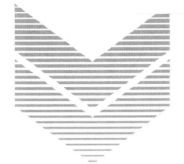

# FUERZA

---

## A FEMALE'S GUIDE TO
## STRENGTH & PHYSIQUE

---

BY

**MARISA INDA**

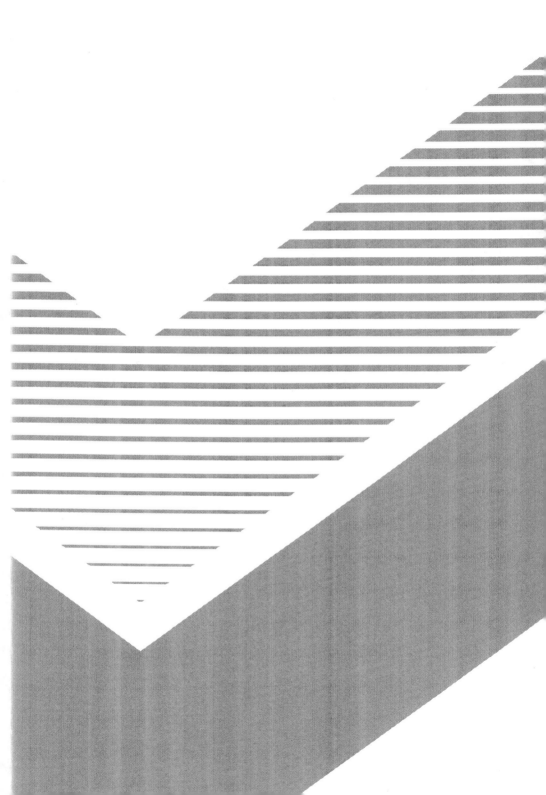

# TABLE OF
# CONTENTS

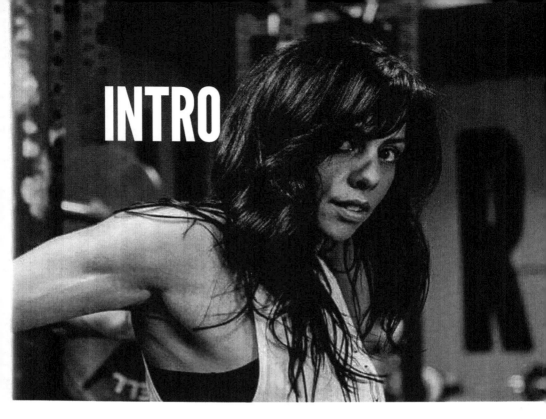

# INTRO

## BACKGROUND

I would like to thank you for taking the time to purchase and read this book. I have been lifting weights for more than half my life, and it gives me so much joy to share what I have learned-- especially since I had to learn by trial and error in the pre-social media age. As I look back at that time, it wasn't exactly trendy to be a female stepping foot into male dominated gyms, and I recognize how important it is to empower other women to do so with more knowledge and less fear than I had.

Let me take a step back, though, and give you a brief glimpse into my background and childhood, so you have a better understanding of what led me into the gym for the first time at 17 years old. I'm pretty fortunate I come from good stock--I like to say I'm strong because of my Sangre. My father is Basque and an immigrant from Spain--if you haven't heard about the Basque stone lifters I suggest you Google it; they are some of the strongest people around, and my Aita is no exception. My mom is Mexican and if there is one thing that speaks volumes about her mental toughness it would have to be that she has had root canals done sans Novocain (interesting side note, like her, all cavities I ever had were also done with no numbing and the mental toughness torch has been passed to my daughter who does the same). One of the most important lessons my

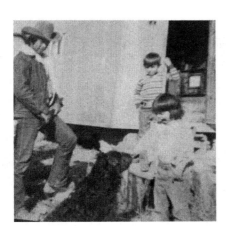

mother taught me was no matter what always tira pa'delante (always go forward). Life throws a lot of curveballs. It's important to always keep moving forward; even if it's at a snail's pace, you're still making progress. This is true not only in life but in lifting where progress takes years and is sometimes measured in small increments (a.k.a. fractional plates).

Growing up on a farm, I spent a lot of time outside, and I was very much a tomboy. I used to jump on-and-off the tailgate of the truck as hay was being unloaded, flipped around on the furniture, and I'd jump from the chicken coop to the tractors nearby--pretty sure I had invented Parkour before it became a thing.  My mom decided to enroll me in gymnastics so I wouldn't hurt myself at home. I instantly fell in love with it, and I'm a huge proponent for every kid being enrolled in tumbling early on because I think it has the best carry over to every other sport. Gymnastics taught me spatial awareness, gave me increased leg, back and shoulder flexibility, explosive power, and increased upper body strength, which many women in strength sports lack. I credit gymnastics for my good technique in lifting today. Unfortunately, it was a very expensive sport, which meant I went on and off and only when we had extra money. My grandpa built me a bar that was attached to the chicken coop and a beam that he made out of 2x4's and carpet. This gave me the opportunity to practice at home when we didn't have the money to attend the gym. My sister used to spot me while doing back flips on this rickety 4 inch carpeted beam, and now that I'm a parent I would be mortified to see my kids doing what we did--it's honestly a miracle no necks were ever broken. An important lesson I learned from this time in my life is, regardless of circumstances, when you're passionate about something you stay consistent the best you can. I also learned that the increased upper body strength gave my brother and

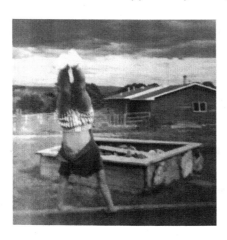

me the ability to hustle his friends and make some extra money betting that I could beat them in arm wrestling and bench competitions-I hope I didn't unknowingly turn these guys into the creepers that now DM women who lift for wrestling rates.

During high school I stuck with gymnastics but knew aiming for the Olympics was not realistic given my age (all elite gymnasts are under 18) and the huge gaps in structured training--not to mention they cut the team my senior year. Since I was accustomed to being active and was looking for something to do, I decided to join the track team. I hated it; however, I gutted it out and lettered because it's not in my nature to quit. But I can say with 100% certainty that running is not for me. I did make some amazing friends during that time, and it was my friend Kendra who invited me to the gym she attended-- which landed me in a step aerobics class. I laugh now, but if it weren't for her and that dreadful class, I never would've ventured down to the weight room.

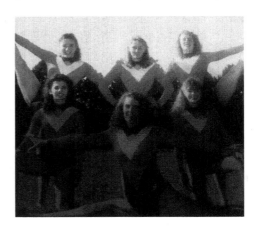

# BODYBUILDING INTRO

Bodybuilding is about creating an illusion: in bodybuilding circles, you'll often hear people say things like "that physique look aesthetically pleasing" or "they have good lines and symmetry." While some people may be genetically blessed with the perfect proportions, the rest of us have to create them. For example, adding size to your shoulders, lats and quads will create the illusion of a smaller waist. Though it is a myth you can spot reduce, you can in fact train lagging areas more frequently and add more size to them.

That first day in the weight room, I had no idea what I was doing. There was no internet back then--no social media gurus with instructional videos. Instead of being a faceless lurker behind a screen, I was forced to be a world class creeper in person. I saw a girl who I thought had an amazing physique and quite frankly I wanted to look like her. She had big legs, a small waist, and developed shoulders--I identified with her body type since gymnastics left me looking more muscular than other girls my age.  For the first time, I looked at my legs and felt proud that

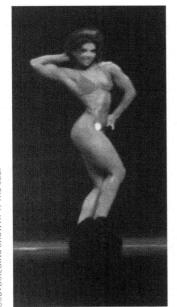

they were "thick." Like any good creeper, instead of talking to her, I just watched what she did and would follow her around the gym doing every exercise she had just finished doing. These days we have it good; Instagram allows us to follow people without the risk of a restraining order.

After a few weeks of shadowing this girl, I discovered Flex magazine (the bodybuilding bible in the 90s) and found some training partners who knew a lot more than me. I was very fortunate to be surrounded by people who trained smart by incorporating compound movements first: Squat, Bench, and Deadlift with the accessory work completed afterward and using free weights rather than machines whenever possible. We did body part splits and a typical week would look something like:

**MONDAY:** Chest / Triceps
**TUESDAY:** Legs / Quad Focus
**WEDNESDAY:** Back / Biceps
**THURSDAY:** Off
**FRIDAY:** Shoulders / Chest
**SATURDAY:** Legs / Hamstring & Glute Focus

During this time there were a lot of drop sets, giant sets, supersets and burnout sets (now called AMRAPS) involved. The weight used was not always maximal but involved a lot more volume--which

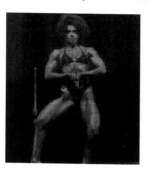

by no means meant we used the same weight week after week. The goal in bodybuilding is to put on more muscle, which requires adding more weight to the bar while keeping volume higher; this is what leads to increased strength and a better overall physique.

The main difference in the compound movements that differentiate bodybuilding from powerlifting are:

### SQUATS

During my bodybuilding days, squats were high bar only and with a more narrow stance than what is typically seen in powerlifting (although recently I decided a more narrow stance was also optimal for my low bar work). Highbar lends itself to a more upright body position and therefore makes the quads work harder--plus we all wanted to squat like Frank Zane.

### BENCH PRESS

Unlike powerlifting, with bodybuilding, there is minimal arch, more of an elbow flare and sometimes even partial reps. Feet can be up on the bench and is primarily touch n go.

### DEADLIFTS

I rarely did sumo during my bodybuilding days since deads were done on a back day and conventional lifting is more back intensive.

Since it was a lot more rep work, I typically wore straps, and there was a lot more rack pulls during this time since rack pulls eliminate the leg drive and make the low back work harder.

Adjustments would be made to focus on any lagging bodyparts; if it needed more size, it would just be trained more frequently. The great part about starting out this way is that I was building a solid foundation because nothing was being neglected. I wasn't pushing crazy heavy weight all the time. I was putting on muscle while staying injury free, and this slower progression also allowed my tendons and ligaments to get strong along the way. I didn't know it then, but I was in a very long hypertrophy block. Another bonus, because I was young and unable to afford a trainer or nutritionist, I was discovering what worked and what didn't work for ME, and how training and proper nutrition could lead to beautiful physique changes.

*"Every block of stone has a statue inside of it, and it is the task of the sculptor to discover it."* — Michelangelo

I competed frequently in bodybuilding those first few years placing first in the teen division at all meets (probably because there weren't many teen girls lifting weights back then) and holding my own in the open division placing in the top 5 at most shows and 6th at the Jr. USA's. I enjoyed competing and the challenge of improving my physique, but I also knew that it was headed in a direction I was not willing to go in regards to the muscularity of the women and the prevalent use of steroids. I continued to train but focused on getting my degree and eventually starting a family.

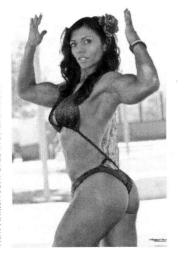

THIS IS THE LAST PHYSIQUE COMPETITION THAT MARISA COMPETED IN 2012 AT AGE 36.

And in case you're wondering, I did eventually talk to the girl whose physique I admired so much; she gave me diet advice and informed me, my boyfriend at the time, was hitting on her and I deserved better--she was right.

Here are some of my favorite bodybuilding strategies and exercises to develop each bodypart.

## INTENSITY TECHNIQUES

### DROP SETS
Technique where you perform a set to near failure, reduce the weight and repeat.

### GIANT SETS
Four or more exercises that target the same muscle group performed back to back with minimal rest.

### SUPERSETS
Two exercises done back to back that target different muscle groups (antagonist - chest and back) or two exercises done back to back that target the same muscle group (Agonist - triceps pushdowns superset with dips).

### BURNOUT SETS / AMRAPS
Perform an exercise until failure (No longer able to maintain form).

# EXERCISES

## BACK
- Lat Pulldowns
  - Front / Behind Neck
- DB / Barbell Bentover Rows
- Chest Supported Rows
- Seated Rows
- Pendlay Rows
- Single Arm DB Rows
- Pullovers
- Back Raises
- Pull-Ups

## SHOULDERS
- Military Press
  - Standing / Seated / Single Arm / DB / Barbell
- Side Laterals
  - Standing / Seated
- Front Raises DB / Plate
- Bent Over Laterals

## BICEPS
- Curls (Hammer, EZ-Curl Bar, Preacher Curls, 21's)
- Chin-Ups

## TRICEPS
- Pushdowns
- Kickbacks
- Palms-In DB Press
- Skullcrushers
- Dips

## CHEST ACCESSORIES
- Incline Barbell Press
- Flat / Incline DB Press
- Flat / Incline DB Fly
- Cable Crossovers
- Chest Press Machine
- Push-Ups

## ABS
- Leg Raises
- Planks
- Standard Crunches

## HAMSTRINGS
- RDL's
- Leg Curls
- Single Leg Curls
- Hip Thrusters
- Glute Ham pull throughs
- GHR

## CALVES
- Calf Raises
  - Standing / Leg Press
- Donkey Raises

## QUADS
- Leg Press
- Hack Squats
- Reverse Hacks
- Lunges
- Step Ups
- Leg Extensions

# TRAINING WHILE PREGNANT

Training with a baby bump wasn't as en vogue as it seems to be nowadays. I can remember all the looks I would get from other gym members and comments about how I was going to hurt my baby--my parenting was being judged before I even had my child. I talked to my doctor, and since I had no complications and had been consistently working out, I could continue training; I just needed to listen to my body and stop if anything felt abnormal. I trained the entire time during both of my pregnancies; it made labor easier and made me feel like I wasn't entirely losing my identity, which is important when you're used to being in shape, active and your body is going through a ton of changes. I wasn't trying to set any world records or get leaner; training while pregnant was for me about maintenance and preserving the muscle I had worked so hard to get.

Here's a quick look at how my training was during each trimester and what considerations need to be made as your belly grows.

## CONSIDERATIONS FOR TRAINING WHILE PREGNANT

### FIRST TRIMESTER

Most women don't find out they're pregnant until they are about 8-9 weeks in, so nothing really changes-your caloric intake is also unchanged. You may feel more tired and possibly have morning sickness, but for most of us, it looks pretty similar to pre-pregnancy. For me, this meant I was still training like normal: bodybuilding style 4-5 days a week, which included squatting, benching and deadlifting. Since I didn't start powerlifting until after I had kids, my rep ranges were still high and the weight loads were submaximal, and if I felt tired or sick, I just scaled back my workout.

## SECOND TRIMESTER

This is the time where others notice you're pregnant and you start to see the outward physical changes as your belly grows. If you experienced morning sickness, this is hopefully the trimester where it subsides. I was still able to comfortably train the same as my first trimester, and my caloric intake only increased by about 300 calories. No movements bothered me. I did, however, stop using my belt because I found it to be too restricting around my stomach. Typically exercises, like bench pressing, that require you to be on your back are uncomfortable as the belly grows. If benching is a no go, substitute chest press machine or incline DB work. There is always a work around that will let you target the same muscle groups without causing you discomfort. Listen to your body: we are all going to be different when it comes to training during pregnancy. Just because I was able to bench press safely doesn't mean you should--when in doubt, avoid it.

## THIRD TRIMESTER

Is this pregnancy thing over yet? For most of us, this is when we feel the most uncomfortable and the belly is really making our shirts work hard--caloric intake only increased about 100 calories from the 2nd trimester to 400. I was still able to train four times a week, but I did have to make some exercise adjustments. Common exercises that I avoided were anything that put me on my stomach, such as lying leg curls. Squats were done with a much wider stance and I switched to sumo pulls to make room for my baby belly. Again, I wasn't going heavy, and I scaled back on the volume on the days I felt tired.

Not going to lie and say it was all peachy, I had to take it day by day and modify as I went. There were times when I felt sick and more tired than usual, there was also that one time I ate a habanero stuffed olive and almost went into labor, but I was also creating a beautiful little life. Nine months go by so fast and with proper nutrition and continued activity, you won't lose that hard earned muscle you worked so hard for pre-baby. The body is amazing at bouncing back, and you'd be surprised at how quickly your strength returns as well.

## TRAINING EXPECTATIONS DURING AND AFTER PREGNANCY

I remember after my first child was born thinking it was going to be business as usual, I couldn't have been more wrong. Adjusting to a new person in the mix was really difficult. My daughter had severe colic, cried non-stop, and didn't sleep through the night until she was three years old--at times I was so tired I'm not sure if she or I cried more.

I gained roughly 20 pounds with both of my pregnancies, and I remember after my first child being really upset because I could literally pull the skin on my stomach like a rubber band, except it didn't snap back. I cried thinking a flat, tight stomach was a thing of the past. On the one hand, you're in awe of this new little life you're holding, and on the other hand you feel like your body has just betrayed you. As with most things in life you have to be patient--the body is miraculous and even though there are changes (maybe a few stretch marks here and there) things do return to normal.

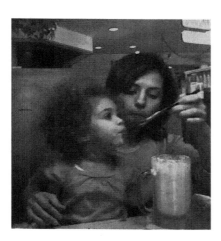

Training postpartum is really important whether you're on baby number 1 or juggling multiple kids. It's easy to lose ourselves, get consumed with parenting and feel selfish for wanting to escape to the gym for an hour, but it's a much-needed sanity break. For me, training postpartum included some scheduling tweaks as well as expectation management.

## TRAINING POSTPARTUM / THINGS TO KEEP IN MIND BEFORE YOU BEGIN

### AB SEPARATION / DIASTASIS RECTI
Make sure your doctor checks for belly muscle separation before returning to any abdominal work. You can also self-

check at home by Googling "self-check for Diastasis Recti"-
The reason for this is many traditional ab exercises like
planks and crunches can make the separation worse.

### PELVIC FLOOR ISSUES

Pregnancy can sometimes cause the pelvic floor to become
very weak. This means that straining via heavy lifting can
lead to urinary incontinence. For this reason, it's important to
take it slow, do pelvic floor exercises and don't jump right into
heavy lifting.

### NATURAL CHILDBIRTH

If you've given birth naturally postpartum hip change is a real
thing. Our hips were designed to expand to allow the baby
to pass through the canal. It's ok you adapt and your squat
technique will too.

### C-SECTION

If you've had a c-section, your recovery will take longer
because of the major abdominal surgery that took place.
Again, patience will have to be your friend because you will
need to recover this typically takes 6-8 weeks.

### TAKE IT SLOW

Don't walk in the gym your first day expecting to squat your
1 rep max for reps. You've been lifting submaximally for nine
plus months--it'll take some time to feel like your former self,
so be patient.

I went about my training postpartum in trimesters--I figured it
took nine months to make this baby and it would probably take
me around nine plus months to feel like my pre-baby self. Here
is how I went about it:

## FIRST THREE MONTHS POSTPARTUM

After you give birth, everything feels out of place, and your body
just doesn't feel stable. Ligaments that allowed the pelvis girdle
to soften so the baby could pass through the birth canal aren't
firm yet. Your uterus can take up to 8 weeks to return to its
normal size and aside from all the body changes, lack of sleep
with a newborn can make you feel like a zombie. For this reason,
I didn't return to the gym until about three weeks postpartum,

and my workouts were very easy and consisted of light, full body, DB workouts, three times a week. I avoided heavy lifting during this time to give my body time to heal internally and wasn't doing any barbell squatting, benching and deadlifting, but I was moving and getting to know my body again. My workouts were also very quick; they lasted 30-40 minutes at most--mainly because my daughter cried so much that it was very hard to find anyone to watch her. I'm glad I didn't rush things because I didn't have urinary incontinence issues before kids and I haven't peed the platform while deadlifting post kids--I stayed patient and of course did a million Kegels.

## THREE TO SIX MONTHS POSTPARTUM

By this time you're more in a routine, and you may be back at work as well. I had a 9-5 corporate job which meant I really had to prioritize my time--sometimes I would even train during my lunch hour so I could get it done. I added in light barbell work but kept to my full body workout routine. These were volume intensive and because I was limited by the time it had a great cardio effect as well. I trained about 4-5 times per week depending on my schedule and how my body was feeling.

### FULL BODY SAMPLE ROUTINE

BARBELL SQUAT: 12-15 reps
BENT-OVER ROW: 12 reps (separate bar set up with different weight)
PUSH-UPS: 12
CRUNCHES: 12
REST 2 MINUTES
REPEAT 6x

Full body workouts are great because you hit everything and you are only limited by your imagination. There are many ways to put together quick and effective routines that are challenging as hell.

## SIX TO NINE MONTHS POSTPARTUM

By this time I was really starting to feel more stable and like my old self. I returned to my body part split training and started increasing the intensity weight wise. I wasn't breastfeeding past three months, so I didn't have to worry about decreased milk supply. If you are breastfeeding just make sure you are taking in enough calories to compensate for the increased activity. I think it's important to remember that everyone's journey is going to be different. Some women regain their shape much faster, have no stretch marks, and it's like pregnancy never happened. Meanwhile, for some, it's a much longer process. Be patient, don't compare yourself to others, be kind to your postpartum body, and above all be consistent.

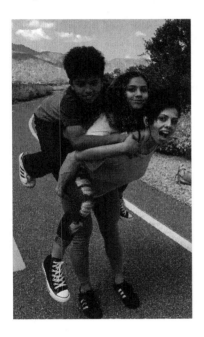

Being a mom has only motivated me to be better. I am stronger today than I was pre-kids, I am competing against the best in the world as an elite powerlifter, and I even got my abs back. My kids are happy, well adjusted and are seeing firsthand the importance of being active and staying healthy.

Moms and moms-to-be, you are still RELEVANT, DESIRABLE and CAPABLE of being more. You can still set PRs in the gym and at home. My competitive journey didn't end after having kids; I just added to my cheering section.

# TRANSITION TO
# POWERLIFTING

I really wanted to compete again, so my training had more purpose and an end goal, but bodybuilding just didn't appeal to me anymore. I had always been fairly strong so when I stumbled upon a flyer for a powerlifting meet, I didn't even think twice and just entered. I remember feeling the same way I did at 17 years old during my first bodybuilding meet; not 100% prepared but soaking in the experience, having fun and learning as much as I could from the other competitors. I had still trained bodybuilding style at this point so my day didn't end with any world records being smashed but I absolutely fell in love with it. Unlike bodybuilding, where the judging could be very subjective, in powerlifting, you were either strong enough to lift the weight on the bar, or you weren't. All I could think about was how could I get better and how do I change what I'm doing in the gym to increase my total at my next meet. I read as much as I could and changed my training from body part splits to linear periodization that included two upper days and two lower days-just like in my bodybuilding days trying to figure out what was working and what wasn't as I went along.

# MY FIRST MEET

When I did my first meet, I had no idea what to expect. I had never been to a powerlifting meet, but I knew I had decent strength and wanted to compete in something. Unlike, a lot of people I talk to today about competing, I didn't look up numbers to see if I would be good enough or competitive (I wasn't even familiar with the rules), I simply showed up the day of the meet just wanting to have fun and enjoy the experience.

During equipment check, I was told my lifting belt did not meet the requirement because it was a leather bodybuilding belt which was too wide in the back. Thankfully, we had a razor blade, and we were able to shave the back down so it would pass. In the rules briefing I would learn that the bench had to be paused, which is also something I hadn't trained for at the time. I think because I didn't have any set expectations these sort of hiccups didn't even phase me, I knew that I just needed to make due. I was still squatting high bar, no knee sleeves, benching with very minimal arch, and wore my old Chuck Taylors for every single lift--I was also starving the entire day because I had no food and didn't realize it would take more than an hour to do three lifts.

This meet stands out as one of my most memorable ones because this is where I fell in love with the idea of getting stronger. I didn't set any world records, in fact, I think I went 4/9 this day and who knew that this would be the defining moment that would change the course of my life and take me around the world competing.

I was progressing, but something was missing--I even had a meet where I bombed out and missed lifts entirely. I needed a second pair of eyes and someone more experienced than myself--so I turned my programming over to Chad Wesley Smith.

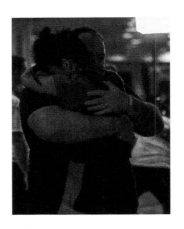

Here's a quick snapshot of my meet numbers from the time I programmed myself until now under CWS:

| DATE | MEET | BW | SQUAT | BENCH | DEAD | TOTAL |
|------|------|------|------|------|------|------|
| 08/11 | Cal State Games | 114lbs | 225lbs | 132lbs | 303lbs | 660 |
| 11/11 | SoCal Regionals | 112lbs | 248lbs | 154lbs | 341lbs | 743 |
| 08/12 | Raw Nats (BOMBED OUT) | 110lbs | 0 | 0 | 0 | 0 |
| 11/12 | SoCal Regionals | 110lbs | 264lbs | 170lbs | 358lbs | 792 |
| 07/13 | Raw Nats (OFF-INJURY) | 109lbs | 264lbs | 170lbs | 325lbs | 760 |
| 02/14 | Arnold Pro Raw | 110lbs | 270lbs | 175lbs | 336lbs | 781 |
| 06/14 | IPF Raw Worlds | 109lbs | 270lbs | 165lbs | 340lbs | 775 |
| 07/14 | Raw Nats | 111lbs | 292lbs | 176lbs | 352lbs | 820 |
| 11/14 | AZ Fall Classic | 110lbs | 303lbs | 187.5lbs | 363lbs | 854 |
| 03/15 | Arnold Pro Raw | 111lbs | 292lbs | 193lbs | 369lbs | 854 |
| 10/15 | Raw Nats (OFF-INJURY) | 112lbs | 297lbs | 187lbs | 370lbs | 854 |
| 03/16 | Arnold Pro Raw | 110lbs | 292lbs | 181lbs | 385lbs | 859 |
| 06/16 | IPF Raw Worlds | 112lbs | 292lbs | 198lbs | 380lbs | 870 |
| 10/16 | Raw Nats | 112lbs | 319lbs | 181lbs | 402lbs | 902 |
| 03/17 | Arnold Grand Prix ALL-TIME TOTAL WORLD RECORD | 114lbs | 330lbs | 204lbs | 413lbs | 948 |
| 06/17 | IPF Raw Worlds WORLD CHAMPION | 112lbs | 314lbs | 209lbs | 402lbs | 925 |

I'm very proud of the progress I was able to make on my own. However, it's been so much fun working with Chad and making improvements at an elite level--where adding to your total takes more work, and more programming thought. One of my favorite memories of this time working together has been breaking the All-Time Total World Record at the 2017 Arnold Grand Prix.

# WORLD RECORD STORY

I've had training blocks with ups and downs, but this particular training block was perfect. I was hitting and at times exceeding all the numbers we had planned for in training. My confidence levels in every lift (especially squat) were very high, and I wasn't even on the radar as someone that could potentially win this meet--I don't mind being the underdog. Every lift went exactly as planned and it was my first 9/9 day. Walking out for that final pull, when that's all that stands between you and the win, and locking it out is the most amazing feeling. On top of setting the all time world record, winning best lifter was just icing on the cake.

This meet was also on the main stage inside the venue for Arnold, which meant we had a huge crowd and the energy was electric. I know Chad gets more nervous for me to compete than I do, but as the lifter, I'm always just as concerned to do well and prove that his programming is the best. I think my favorite part though, is looking at the pictures and seeing that Chad was just as excited and pumped for my lifts as I was.

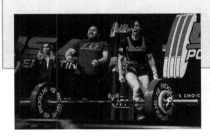
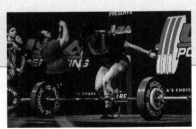

# TRAINING THE SQUAT

## EQUIPMENT

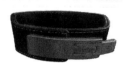

**BELT:** A good belt is a key investment for a serious lifter. I wear an Inzer Forever Lever Tapered Belt. The taper will be more comfortable for shorter females, as it won't dig into the ribs. A 11mm or 13mm belt is appropriate, but the 13mm option may feel too bulky for smaller lifters.

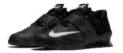

**HEELED SHOES:** Shoes with a heel are particularly useful if you need extra ankle mobility to be able to squat to depth. They are more expensive but are very sturdily built.

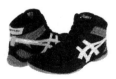

**FLAT SHOES:** I prefer to squat in flat shoes because I have the necessary ankle mobility to squat to depth without a heel and felt the heel was tipping me forward too much. When looking for a good flat shoe, you want a thin and sturdy heel.

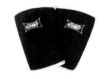

**KNEE SLEEVES:** For general training, Knee Sleeves aren't a must, but as your training volume and weights increase, they are a nice comfort to help keep your knees warm and make you feel a bit more secure.

## TECHNIQUE

Unlike bodybuilding, PL squat technique usually means a lower bar placement on the back-roughly 2-3 inches lower. This may feel odd at first if you've only ever done high bar. However, the leverages with low bar lend itself to a bigger squat. This means

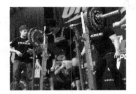

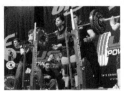

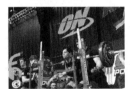

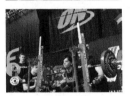

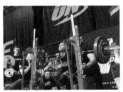

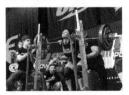

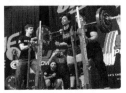

there will be a bit more forward lean versus high bar where you're able to stay more upright.

**1.** A tight upper back is step one to a strong squat setup. Squeeze your shoulder blades together and pull your elbows towards each other slightly behind your back with the bar across your reach delts.

**2.** Set a strong position before you descent by drawing in a big breath, pushing down and out through your obliques into the belt and flexing your glutes and quads. Hold in your air and tight braced core position throughout the lift.

**3.** Initiate the squat by simultaneously bending the knees and hips. Maintain even pressure on your foot between the big toe, little toe and heel as you descend.

**4.** In the bottom of the squat, aka The Hole, the top surface of your hips should be aligned below the top of your knees. Weight should still be evenly distributed throughout your foot, and your knees should be tracking slightly over and in line with your toes.

**5.** As you come out of the hole in the squat, focus on simultaneously pushing with your upper back into the bar, as you keep your knees forward, as near the same position they were in the hole, as possible so you can fully utilize your quad strength.

**6.** Continue to try and accelerate the bar through the top of your lift, creating equal force with your back into the bar, as with your feet into the floor.

**7.** Maintain balance in the top of the lift with quads and glutes flexed as hard as possible. If you are doing multiple reps, this is the time to take another breath in and brace your core.

## SQUAT PROGRAMMING CONSIDERATIONS

Building a strong squat requires one thing above all else, strong legs. Improving the strength of your legs begins with building their size, particularly the quads. Training for size, also known as Hypertrophy Training, is driven by increasing volume up to your body's tolerance. When training for Hypertrophy, we want to train in the following ranges:

- 60-75% of your 1rm
- 6-12 reps per set
- 15-25 sets per week

If you don't currently know your 1rm, the simplest way to find out would to just see how heavy you can go with good technique for 1 to 5 reps. If you do more than 1 rep, you can find your projected max by using:

(Weight x Reps x 0.0333) + Weight = Projected Max

These 15-25 sets per week can be made up of several different exercises, but prioritizing exercises that target the quads well and lend themselves to higher volumes are important. Some of my favorite exercises to build leg size and strength are, in order of usefulness:

- High Bar Squat
- Front Squat
- Belt Squat
- Leg Press / Hack Squat
- Walking Lunges
- Split Squats
- Step Ups

Figuring out how many sets you should be doing each week will rely on trial and error but the 15-25 sets/week should be a good guide but make sure to allow yourself to start on the lower side of the range, or even slightly below it, so that you can build up over time. The frequency of squatting (how many times per week you're doing it) will vary based on your fitness, experience, size, strength and of course, schedule, but 2-3x/week is what I've found to work best for me. If you are a total beginner, try starting at 2x/week and then as you become more fit for squatting, you

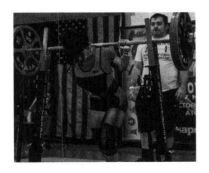

can try increasing to 3x and potentially even 4x in a single week but keep in mind that the total weekly volume is the most significant factor.

The length of time you spend in a Hypertrophy phase for squats will vary based on the same factors as frequency. If you are preparing for a powerlifting meet and have less than five years of serious training experience, I'd suggest you spend up to 50% of your time in Hypertrophy training; this could be the first six weeks of a 12-week meet prep cycle. If you don't have a meet planned or are just training to improve your physique, you can spend as long as four months training for Hypertrophy. Remember that Hypertrophy is part of the long game, it isn't about necessarily getting stronger right now; it is about setting you up for long term success. Hypertrophy training, besides growing the size of your muscles and with that, their potential strength; it will also improve your work capacity so you can do more quality work throughout the rest of the training cycle-which in turns means your physique changes.

Once you've spent the necessary time building up the size of your legs, now it is time to improve their strength. Strength Training is best achieved in the following ranges:

75-90% of your 1rm
3-6 reps per set
8-16 sets per week

As you progress into Strength Training, you'll need to choose exercises that are better suited for using more weight and are more specific to your competition lifts. My favorite squat variations for Strength Training are:

Low Bar Squat
High Bar Squat
Pause Squat
Front Squat
Belt Squat

Exercises like Leg Press/Hack Squat and single leg work can still have some usefulness, especially for more beginner lifters, but they shouldn't be your priority.

Strength Training is about adding more weight to the bar each week, so volume will need to decrease with time so that you can recover properly. Start conservatively on each training cycle; this will give you room to improve because training too heavy, too frequently will be too difficult to recover from.

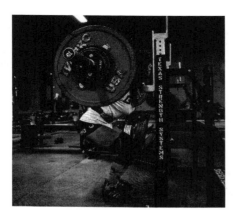

Since Strength Training requires heavier weights, it is more stressful to your body (muscles/joints) and nervous system; generally, this means you can't train for it as long. For powerlifting, most women (except the very experienced ones) will need to spend 20-40% of their time on it, that would likely be 3-4 weeks out of a 12-week meet prep cycle. If you're training for physique, strength training is still important as it will help you use heavier weights during your next training cycle (which will help build more muscle) and re-sensitive your body for higher volumes. The longest time you'll likely want to spend in Strength Training is three months but as short as three weeks can be effective.

If you're preparing for a Powerlifting meet or just looking to test your strength and push your biggest weights, Peaking Training is the next phase you'll go through. Peaking Training is the heaviest and most specific aspect of training for max strength. During Peaking you'll train in these ranges:

90%+ of your 1rm
1-3 reps per set
4-8 sets per week

Peaking Training is the most taxing on your nervous system, so

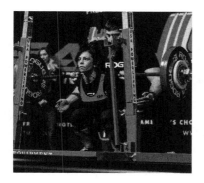

volume is inherently low. Since it is right before you compete or test your 1rm, you need to focus nearly all your attention to your competition technique in the squat, any variations you use beyond that will be very minimal.

Female lifters will have a very short peaking phase, particularly as beginners. Since women lack the same testosterone levels as their male counterparts, they will lose muscle much faster, and since Peaking Training is inherently low volume, it can lead to muscle loss if done for too long. Peaking training for female lifters should range from 1-3 weeks.

Training at above 90% of your 1rm is the most neurally taxing and neural recovery takes longer than muscular recovery, so your hard training will be less frequent during this phase, maybe only 1-2x/week. Because perfecting technique is such a high priority in this time, you may want to add 1-2 more sessions (after your benching or on off days) where you do 60-70% in the squat from 3-8 sets of 1 rep while having great focus on your technique (which you should always have).

Building bigger, stronger legs and a heavier squat is the foundation of a great physique AND success on the powerlifting platform.

# TRAINING
# THE BENCH

## EQUIPMENT

**WRIST WRAPS:** I don't personally wear wrist wraps while benching and think that it is useful, particularly at lighter weights, to train without them so you can build up the strength of your joints. If you feel comfortable with them in competition feel free to use them. If you are struggling with wrist pain in the bench press, they can be useful as well.

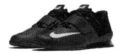

**SHOES:** A flat or heeled shoe, similar to what you wear in the squat, is appropriate for the bench press too. You want to be stable and able to keep your whole foot on the ground throughout the lift.

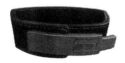

**BELT:** Some lifters choose to wear a belt for the bench press for added tightness and support, I do not wear one and can't really comment on their usefulness here.

## TECHNIQUE

1. A good setup with pressure on your feet, our shoulder blades retracted, and weight up on your traps is critical to maximizing your bench press.

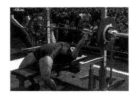

2. Squeeze the bar hard in your hands throughout the lift to increase tension throughout your body. Draw a big breath in before bringing the bar down and hold that breath in throughout the rep.

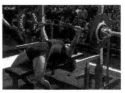

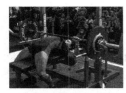
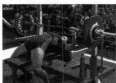
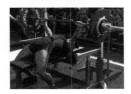

**3.** Focus on keeping your chest as high as possible as you bring the bar down to your chest. Where you touch on the chest will vary slightly based on your setup and leverages but a consistent touch point is key. This will likely mean that your elbows are around a 45-degree angle from your body.

**4.** Drive your toes into the end of your shoes as you initiate the press, this will create leg drive and help you stay tight.

**5.** Accelerate the bar through to lockout. The bar path should resemble a 'j' pattern, moving from your chest towards your face and up. Hold the bar with your triceps flexed hard at lockout.

## BENCH PROGRAMMING CONSIDERATIONS

The bench press is often a frustration for female lifters, but with patience and consistency you will improve. Females lag behind in the bench press compared to their male counterparts because of a relative lack of upper body muscle mass; during Hypertrophy Training, we will combat that problem. I have been able to become one of the best female bench pressers in the World, and I have my 20+ years of bodybuilding training to thank for it. You can arch all you want and take the widest grip possible, but if you don't build muscle in your chest, triceps, shoulders and upper back, your bench press will never be what it could. Hypertrophy Training for the Bench Press should be done in the following ranges:

> 65-80% of your 1rm
> 6-12 reps per set
> 20-30 sets per week

The bench press can generally tolerate the highest volumes of training and female lifters tend to be able to handle more sets at relatively higher intensities than male lifters. Your 20-30 work sets directed at improving the bench press each week should include, in order of usefulness:

Competition Grip Bench Press
Wide Grip Bench Press
Close Grip Bench Press
Incline Bench Press
Standing Military Press
DB Pressing (Flat, Incline, Decline, Military)
Push Ups (Weighted If You Can)
Flyes (Dumbbell and Machine)
Machine Chest Press
Skullcrushers
Tricep Pushdowns

I can't emphasize the value of pushups enough for the beginner and even intermediate female lifters. Push-ups have always been a big part of my training, whether that was challenging my brother's friends to pushup contests, using them during gymnastics warm-ups or having fun with my 'pushup flows,' they've been a great contributor to my upper body strength.

Training frequency for the upper body will be a trial and error process as it is for the squat but since the muscles of the upper body are smaller, and the weights you're lifting with them are lighter, you can train them more often. Training for the bench press can often be done 3-5x/week for female lifters. Keep in

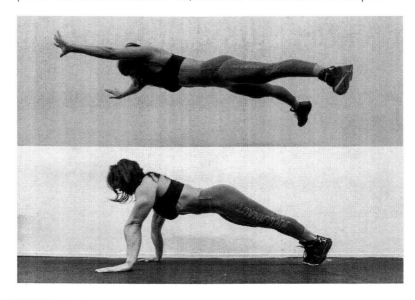

mind that not all of these sessions will be as much volume as you can handle but some undulation of harder and easier days would be appropriate.

Hypertrophy training for the bench press should make up an even greater proportion of your training time than either the Squat or Deadlift does. Spending up to 66% of your bench press training in Hypertrophy Training could be useful, this will give you ample time to build muscle. Hopefully, if you're reading this book, you aren't concerned about getting 'too bulky,' I would be hard pressed to find a serious female lifter who feels like they add upper body muscle mass easily.

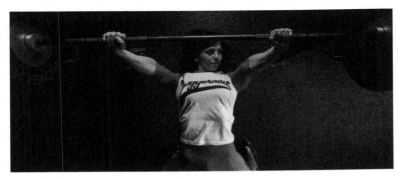

Once you have dedicated sufficient time to building up the size of your chest, shoulders, and arms, you can now add more intensity with Strength Training:

  80-92.5% of your 1rm
  3-6 reps per set
  15-20 sets per week

Bench Press training generally doesn't offer as much variation as Squats or Deadlifts do, but you should focus your exercise selection a bit more towards movements that allow you to use heavier weights:

  Competition Grip Bench Press
  Wide Grip Bench
  Close Grip Bench
  Spoto Press
  Bench w/ Slingshot or Reverse Bands

Standing or Seated Military Press
DB Pressing (Flat, Incline, Decline, Military)
Push Ups (Weighted If You Can)
Flyes (Dumbbell and Machine)
Machine Chest Press
Skullcrushers
Tricep Pushdowns

I still included the accessory work here because accessory movements are of particular importance for females striving to build a better bench press as well as overall physique development. These smaller movements should be used as a compliment to the bigger exercises; but make sure that once you've done all you feel you can on the primary work, fill in the gaps with smaller exercises that give more focused attention to muscles that may be lagging.

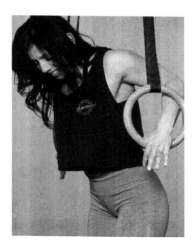

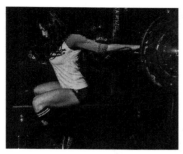

Female lifters can generally do much more volume at relatively heavier weights than male lifters. It wouldn't be uncommon for a female lifter to be able to perform 90%x5 reps in the bench press or multiple sets of 85%x5, while a male lifter may set a five rep max at 85%. Because of this, females need to push the amount of work they're doing during a strength phase, both the volume will be higher as well as the relative intensity. Since most females will only need a very short peaking block for the bench press; spending 30-50% of your training energy in Strength Training is a good strategy.

If you're preparing for a Powerlifting meet or just looking to test your strength and push your biggest weights, Peaking Training is the next phase you'll go through. Peaking Training is the heaviest and most specific aspect of training for max strength. During Peaking you'll train in these ranges:

92.5%+ of your 1rm
1-3 reps per set
6-10 sets per week

Bench 2-3x per week in the above volume/intensity ranges would be good for most during peaking, along with the potential addition of a day that resembles a lighter Strength Training day to ensure that weekly volume stays high and you retain muscle through peaking into the meet.

One great piece of advice I can give to any female lifters looking to improve their bench press is to invest in a set of fractional plates. If the smallest weights you have are 2.5 pounds or 1.25kg, you'll be extremely limiting yourself in the increments of improvement you can make. Being able to make incremental jumps in weight will help bench press strength improve while keeping frustration at bay.

If you are a woman looking for a better bench, put your attention towards building muscle, along with mastering your technique. Know that progress may be slow but with your diligence and perseverance, improvements will come.

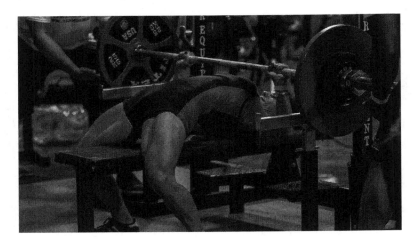

# TRAINING
# THE DEADLIFT

## EQUIPMENT

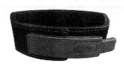

**BELT:** Just like in the squat, a good belt is a worthwhile investment. I wear the same belt for the deadlift as I do for the squat.

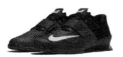

**SHOES:** Thin soled, flat shoes are optimal for the deadlift. I wear wrestling shoes since they grip the floor really well and provide a bit of ankle support as well.

**SOCKS:** Knee high socks are mandatory for competition but I usually wear them during training to help protect my shins, plus they look cute.

## TECHNIQUE

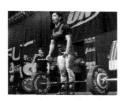

**1.** Your deadlift stance should be the same width that you would do a vertical jump from, right under your hips with your toes straight ahead or slightly turned out. The bar should be aligned over your midfoot, where the knot in your shoelaces is, is a good rule of thumb.

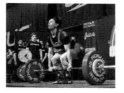

**2.** Hinge your hips down into the start position. Imagine creating a window with your arms and the bar and then putting your knees through that window, your shins should be lightly touching the bar. Generate lat

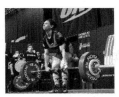

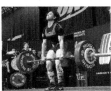

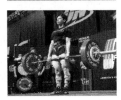

tightness by squeezing your triceps into your lats, as if you are trying to stop someone from tickling your armpits.

3. Drive your feet through the floor, as you pull up and back through the shoulders. As the bar reaches your knees, your shins should have moved into a totally vertical position.

4. As the bar passes your knees, flex your glutes hard to begin extending your hips to meet the bar at lockout.

5. At lockout, stand tall with your quads and glutes flexed as hard as possible. Leave your shoulders as relaxed as possible, so that your arms hang low.

## DEADLIFT PROGRAMMING CONSIDERATIONS

The Deadlift is usually the lift that comes most naturally to female lifters and is a great tool to build strength and muscle throughout the body. Something important to keep in mind with the Deadlift is that it is the most stressful to the body of the three powerlifts, so it needs to be trained the most carefully to ensure progress and avoid overtraining or injury.

When using the Deadlift for Hypertrophy Training, put your focus more on building the muscles needed to have a big deadlift, rather than actually performing lots of heavy deadlifts, this will be particularly true for Sumo Deadlifters. Conventional Deadlifts will generally be better strength builders, even though the Sumo Deadlift may allow you to better express that strength. Too many female lifters seem to automatically think they need to be Sumo Deadlifters but putting in the effort on hard Conventional Deadlift training will yield benefits no matter your style of pulling, as well as building lots of great muscle in the Hamstrings, Glutes and through the entire back.

When training the Deadlift for Hypertrophy, train in the following ranges:

60-75% of your 1rm
6-10 reps per set
15-22 sets per week

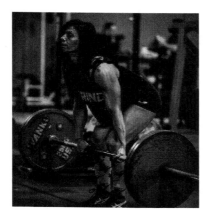

Because Deadlifts from the floor can be so stressful to the body and nervous system, I encourage you to remember that Hypertrophy Training is about building Muscle, you'll have plenty of time before competition to hone your technique. While Conventional Deadlifts from the floor will be the best way to build muscle for the Deadlift, you should focus on the following:

Conventional Deadlift
2-4" Block Pulls or Rack Pulls
RDLs / Box Deadlifts
Good Mornings
Sumo Deadlifts
Deficit Deadlifts
Back Raises
GHRs

When you are using exercises like RDLs and Good Mornings, it is easy to get caught up in the weight you are using but try to make your technique very strict so that you can get the greatest training effect from the lightest weights. If you aren't feeling the muscles working that you're trying to develop, drop the weight and ensure that you're executing them properly.

Deadlift training is the most stressful to the body in every way, so it will require the least amount of training relative to the three lifts. I utilize 1 main deadlift workout per week with 1 secondary workout two days later, 2-3 Deadlift workouts per week, with one of them being significantly lighter should be sufficient.

Hypertrophy Training will be a shorter portion of your training for the Deadlift, as Females are generally more muscular in the areas needed for heavy deadlifting. Even during Hypertrophy Training, I usually use slightly lower reps for the Deadlift than the Squat or Bench Press. If I'm using sets of 10 in the Squat, I will usually do 8s in the Deadlift. Normally, spending 25-40% of your training time on Hypertrophy for the Deadlift.

After you've built up bigger hamstring, glutes and spinal erectors, you're ready to move to Strength Training and improving the force production of those muscles, as well as becoming more specific about your technique.

Strength Training for the Deadlift should done in the following ranges:

   75-90% of your 1rm
   3-5 reps per set
   10-15 sets per week

Strength Training means that you are closer to competition or testing your max in the gym, so developing your technique becomes more of a priority, that needs to be considered when choosing exercises:

   Competition Deadlifts (Conventional or Sumo)
   Conventional Deadlifts (Worth doing even if you compete Sumo)
   3" Competition Block Pulls
   RDLs / Box Deadlifts
   Good Mornings

Accessory work like Back Raises and GHRs are still useful and should be included but aren't specific enough to count towards your 10-15 sets per week.

Training the deadlift hard is great and important to success but as I've become more advanced, I find more and more than stopping 1 rep shy of what I can do is very useful for keeping me healthy and ensuring I can properly recover. With that in mind, don't let your technique deteriorate for an extra rep or 10 extra pounds, pull every rep with great intent toward your technique and as explosively as possible.

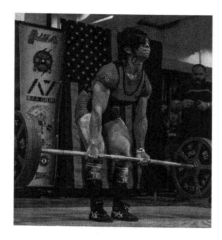

Your strength training will be the bulk of your Deadlift training, taking up 30-60% of your training time.

Pulling a max Deadlift is one of the most empowering feelings you can have as a lifter and Peaking is the time to make that happen. Peaking is about perfecting your technique and preparing your nervous system for max weights, take note that I wrote 'preparing' because too often I see people doing their heaviest deadlifts in training, rather than competition when it counts. During peaking, train your deadlift in the following ranges:

90%+ of your 1rm
1-2 reps per sets
3-5 sets per week

Deadlifting hard, within the parameters above, 1x/week should be sufficient for Conventional Deadlifters, with a 2nd Technique Day where you perform 3-6 sets of 1 rep at 60-70% of your max.

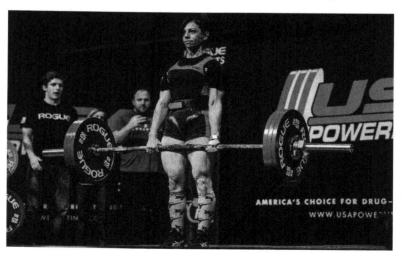

Sumo Deadlift isn't as structurally demanding, so they can likely perform two heavy sessions per week with potentially another Technique Day.

Remember that training is for building your lifts, not testing them, and that holds true for peaking as well. You'll be better off using 5-10 fewer pounds than you may be capable of and ensuring you make all your deadlifts, rather than pushing too far and fatiguing yourself too much in training or damaging your confidence.

Programming for powerlifting can seem overwhelming and if you are a beginner or intermediate lifter, you should seek out a qualified coach but hopefully, this information will help you better understand how well-structured training looks, as well as understanding why you're doing what you're doing.

# STRENGTH AS THE PATH TO AESTHETICS

Strength and aesthetics don't have to be mutually exclusive. The main difference between my own programming and beginning with Chad was, his had more structure and incorporated the different phases (Hypertrophy, Strength, Peaking). In powerlifting, peaking at the right time is crucial. However, for the physique side of things the hypertrophy phase is most important and what adds muscle. This phase mirrored my bodybuilding style volume wise and is why I'm one of the more muscular 52kg lifters in the IPF. Now, this doesn't mean you need to spend ten plus years in this phase as I did; however, it definitely shouldn't be neglected. It takes women much longer than our male counterparts to put on quality muscle--therefore don't be afraid to do 2-3 hypertrophy blocks before jumping into a strength block. Muscle moves weight and the more muscle

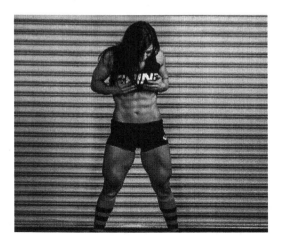

you have, the stronger you will become-- and it's fun when people ask if you're getting ready for a bodybuilding show when you're about to step up on the platform for a powerlifting meet.

Here are a few tips to keep in mind when adding muscle to your frame:

• Don't neglect the accessory exercises. Pick a few basic movements and stick with them for 4-6 weeks. You want to increase strength and proficiency in accessory work too. Don't just go through the motions but really feel the muscles you are working.

• Get your nutrition in order and don't be afraid to fill out your frame. Women tend always to want to cut weight, but if you want to add muscle, you're going to need to eat. Nutrition should match your training block and physique goals. For example, the hypertrophy block is a great time to be in a bulking phase since volume is high and you're going to increase muscle mass in this block. If you are cutting, high volume training is still a good idea because you can eat relatively more and still be in a deficit (high volume training burns more calories) and it will help you retain more muscle.

• Be patient, adding muscle isn't an overnight endeavor. It takes patience, consistency and TIME.

# CALISTHENICS

The day I stepped foot into a weight room I left behind my gymnastics roots and really immersed myself into lifting. Instagram introduced me to people like Frank Medrano and Progressive Calisthenics; they've popularized Urban/Street Calisthenics, which is a combination of classic calisthenics (standard pull-ups) and gymnastics (360 bar spins), and it looked like a lot of fun. I mean what's the point of being strong if you can't move your own bodyweight? I also really missed feeling like I was athletic.

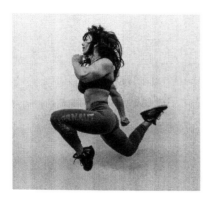

I started incorporating bodyweight movements after my main powerlifting work (mainly on upper days since calisthenics tends to be more upper body intensive in my opinion) and only when I'm in a hypertrophy or strength block. As I get closer to a meet and into my peaking block, where more specificity is required, I stop doing the

explosive floor and bar work. Calisthenics is a whole different rush than lifting weights because it's freestyle and requires a lot more imagination. You'd be surprised how hard it is to move your own bodyweight around, especially to music. It's a pretty badass feeling to still be capable of doing things I did as a 10-year-old gymnast--and let's not forget the social media world loves a good push-up or pull-up flow.

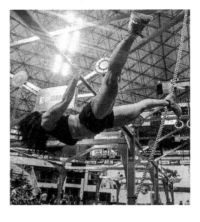

Getting that first-pull up and other quick tips:

• Pull-ups require back strength, mainly in the lats, therefore doing more exercises that will increase strength in this area is essential--Lat Pulldowns, DB rows, Straight arm pull-downs, etc. Make sure you're incorporating these on EVERY upper day. Remember, women can train the upper body with more frequency since these smaller muscles recover much faster.

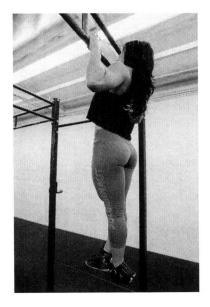

• Dead hangs- A big part of being able to do a pull-up is having the grip strength to hang from the bar. You want to be able to hang with packed shoulders and not feel like your arms are going to detach-- 5-10 second dead hangs after doing lat pull downs is a good way to start increasing your grip strength for that first pull-up.

• Hanging Scapular retraction- Once you feel good about your dead hangs adding in this retraction movement will teach you to engage those lats. From the dead hang position your shoulders will be up by your ears. With your arms straight you want to pull your shoulders down-think about creating distance between your shoulders and ears and keep your chest up-- 3 sets of 8-10 reps after your weight work is ideal.

• Partial Pull-ups- now that you know how to properly engage the lats- from the hanging scapular retraction position just try pulling yourself up towards the bar and don't worry about how far up you can go--even an inch is progress. You'll want to control the negative and repeat. Doing these for a few sets and reps will help you in the bottom portion of the pull-up (which often feels like the hardest part and where people give up).

• Add in progressions- horizontal pull-ups AKA inverted rows, banded pull-ups, jumping pull-ups (jump and get chin over the bar and control the negative) and arm hangs (simply holding your chin above the bar for a few seconds).

• Think about pulling the bar down to you, rather than pulling yourself up to the bar. This should help Lat Pulldowns have a higher carryover to Pull Up strength. What this does is keep your chest up and your elbows behind you. You don't want your elbows to move out in front of you because then you're relying on arm strength over back strength to get you over the bar and the back is much stronger.

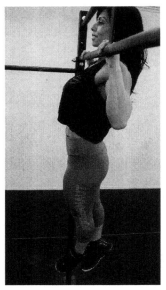

• Focus on staying as tight as possible throughout your body, flex your abs and glutes; this will help you stop from swinging and stay in a better position to allow your lats to work. I like to cross my legs at my ankles to keep my lower half stable.

• If you already have a pull-up and are trying to increase your reps approach it the same way you do strength training-more volume. If you are only able to do two reps, for instance, cut that in half and do more sets. So you'll do 1 rep for eight sets (you've now done eight total reps instead of 2), the following week 1 rep for sets of 10 then, 1 for 12 and so on. After 4-6 weeks you can retest your max pull-ups.

• In lifting, if you want to get better at the lifts and improve your technique you have to practice and the same with pull-ups. The only way to get better is to do them and don't give up-before you know it you'll be air walking to music.

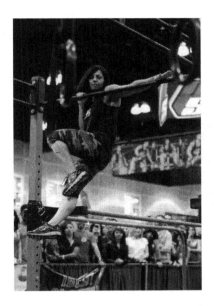

Each one of us has the power to sculpt our bodies and be our own work of art. As more women enter the weight room believing that they are too weak to get that first pull-up or squat two times body weight, it is clear we need to debunk the image of female frailty and solidify our role in the strength world. More often than not women tend to be defined by how "feminine" they can look while putting on muscle. The idea of what femininity and the perfect physique looks like will vary from person to person and it's up to you to define what this looks like for yourself--which often changes as you progress and spend more time in the gym. In this book, my goal is to give you the tools you need to sculpt your physique the way YOU want it while getting stronger in the process. Though our aesthetic goals may differ, we can use similar tools to chisel our bodies the way we want them.

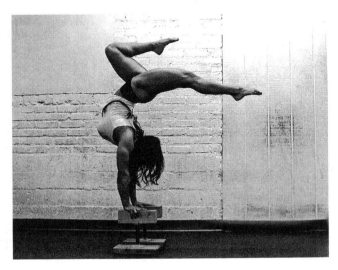

# CARDIO

When you're trying to improve your body composition, weight training alone isn't enough. Conversely, when you're trying to improve your one rep max, cardio is often portrayed as the evil thief of gains. The truth is you can do both with proper balance and prioritizing your goals--and let's face it, having some aerobic capacity comes in handy when you're in a high volume hypertrophy block. The ideal cardio program is going to vary from person to person depending on your goals, preferences, and how much time you have. I do my cardio first thing in the morning at 4:30 a.m. I ride a stationary bike for 30 minutes three times a week on different intervals depending on how I feel. This is the time slot that works for my schedule and is the only time I will actually get it done--I weight train about 6 hours later so there's a sufficient gap. Since my priority is my powerlifting competition schedule, I keep cardio in both hypertrophy and strength blocks and cut it during my peaking block.

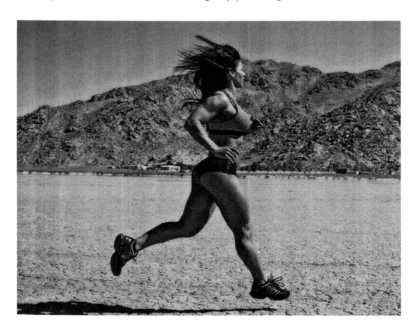

## CARDIO GUIDELINES:

• If you have to combine your resistance training and cardio into one session, do your resistance training first.

• I've found that 2-4 cardio sessions per week for about 20-40 minutes of moderate to intense cardio have no adverse effects on my strength gains, yet help me maintain a comfortable level of leanness.

• HIIT (high intensity) vs. LISS (steady state)- if you've been sedentary for a while high-intensity cardio might be too much too soon. Also, if you're prone to pulling muscles, hill sprints might not be the smartest choice--especially if you haven't done them since your high school track days. Use common sense; low, moderate and intense types of cardio all have their place and can all be effective.

• Pick something you're going to enjoy doing. For most people cardio isn't something they look forward to so if you can't fathom sitting on a bike or walking on a treadmill for 30 minutes, take it outside.

# NUTRITION

I'm not a registered dietitian. The information I present here is based on my own experience and talking with people knowledgeable on the subject.

Nutrition planning and adherence to the plan is the hardest part for most people but will have the biggest impact on displaying the physique you're working so hard to achieve. When I did my first bodybuilding show, I couldn't afford a nutritionist and there weren't all the fancy apps to track macros in those days. The first few years of contest prep for bodybuilding taught me a lot, especially since I was young and on a very tight budget--mainly that your finances don't dictate your food choices.

My approach to dieting has always been, keep it simple and use common sense--it doesn't need to be complicated or expensive. The three main components of any diet are protein, carbohydrates, and fat.

## PROTEIN:
Four calories per gram and can come from animal sources (dairy, eggs, meat, and fish) or plant sources (lentils, beans, soybeans). It's important to eat enough protein if you want to gain and/or maintain muscle, which typically breaks down to 1 gram per pound of lean mass and will make up about 40% of your total caloric intake.

## CARBOHYDRATES:
Four calories per gram and typically broken down into simple (sugars) and complex (starchy) carbs. Carbs have been vilified in a lot of circles but the body uses them as energy and they taste delicious. They fuel our workouts and prevent fatigue by replenishing glucose and glycogen stores. Each individual's intake will vary dependent on activity levels, age, and genetics, but a good starting point is about 40% of your calories coming from carbs--with the simple carbs being utilized best during

training sessions. Keep in mind the optimal percentages for your body and activity level may be different but can be adjusted as you figure out what's working and what's not.

## FATS:

Nine calories per gram and like carbs, fats are given a bad name but they help the body absorb vitamins and keep you satiated longer--which helps you avoid binge eating. Fats like avocados, peanut butter, almond butter, coconut oil, and almonds are great fat sources. Typically 20% of your calories can come from fat. However, if you have high blood pressure you can reduce this percentage and increase the protein and carb percentages. On non-training days I tend to up my fat intake and decrease my carb intake since I'm less active.

Fortunately, there are many apps available so you don't have to do the math and you can quickly calculate what your current caloric maintenance is, however, I prefer that a person track what they're currently eating for about a week. Calorie calculators provide an estimate but, the actual caloric needs will vary from person to person based on a variety of factors--also most people either over or underestimate their activity levels. Tracking for a week will be more accurate (so long as you're honest with yourself) and tell you how much you're currently taking in. Another added benefit of tracking is it gives you a really good peek into your eating habits and may explain why you binge eat, feel fatigued or maybe even feel overly full.

Using myself as an example, as a 5ft 112-116 pound active woman, my maintenance calories are roughly 1300. At my weight and body composition I want to make sure I get at least 90 grams of protein per day, so I aim for a 40,40,20 split-which caps me at 130 grams of protein. Keep in mind that the right macronutrient split for you may be different--some people do better on a higher fart, lower carb, lower protein split. There is flexibility, so if I don't hit the protein requirement or go over a bit on the carbs and fat, there's no need to panic--on none training days I typically reduce my carbs and increase my fat intake. I aim to get as close to the target as possible-progress is key and that means you may not always hit the bullseye. Now, if I wanted to lose weight or go into a cutting phase, I would simply drop my calories, by about 150-200 to start. The mistake a lot of people make is cutting too many calories too soon and that leaves you no room to make adjustments, makes you feel overly hungry and usually results in quitting. Slow and steady wins the race so when you're cutting, cut a few calories out at first and when your weight loss stalls cut a bit more-and be aware of where you're at in your menstrual cycle (temporary weight gain doesn't mean you've stalled). Conversely, if I wanted to go into a massing (bulking) phase, I would add about 150-200 calories and adjust up or down based on how I'm looking. When massing, you will put on a little bit of fat, but there's' no need to put on an excessive amount, therefore, like cutting, I prefer to take it slow and adjust based on my rate of weight gain.

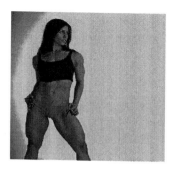

I've moved to a more intuitive eating style, meaning I don't weigh and measure everything out, since I spent years doing that while competing in bodybuilding and I'm pretty good about knowing what my portion sizes look like for my needs. I recently took a day of eating and tracked to see how close I was to my 1300 goal.

Here's what I ate today for example:

## BREAKFAST:
**BLUEBERRY SMOOTHIE** (this is the easiest thing for me in the morning due to a rushed schedule with school drop offs--my kids love it too)
> 1 Cup Oikos Plain Greek yogurt
> ½ Cup frozen blueberries
> Water (amount depends on preferred thickness)
> Two packets of Equal (takes away tartness)
> Blend and enjoy

**225 calories, 21P, 18C, 9F**

## INTRA WORKOUT:
**12OZ GATORADE** (for the quick carbs)
**80 calories, 21C**

## POST TRAINING:
**TERIYAKI BOWL** (4oz of chicken)
- ½ Cup white rice
- ½ Cup steamed broccoli
- 1 Tablespoon of Teriyaki sauce

**326 calories, 40P, 30C, 4F**

## SNACK:
- 1 Green apple
- 1 Tablespoon of peanut butter

**190 calories, 5P, 28C, 8F**

## DINNER:
**CHICKEN VEGETABLE STIR FRY** (a quick and easy favorite)
Add over rice (if you need the carbs)

**240 calories, 23P, 27C, 1F**

## SNACK:
**TWO SCOOPS OF CASEIN PROTEIN**
Mix with a little water (consistency of pudding)

**100 calories, 20P, 4C, 2F**

## TOTAL:
**1161 calories, 109P, 129C, 24F**

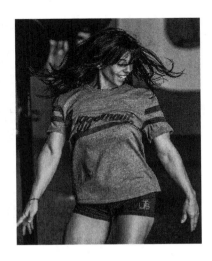

As you can see I was a bit shy meeting my daily caloric values on this day, while on other days I've most likely gone over my goal. I don't eat a perfect diet every single day of my life--it's that on average my food choices balance out.

Realize that we are all different and will have different caloric needs. For example, my training partner Kristen is a 5'5 female who weighs between 145-150lbs.

Her maintenance calories are 2100 and of those calories, her macronutrient percentages are 35p/40c/25f.

Keep in mind you cannot stay in a cutting phase forever and quite frankly who would want to? Each phase is for a specified amount of time-this not only keeps you sane it's how you make the most progress and prevent huge weight fluctuations--three months max per phase is ideal. Once you've come off a cutting or bulking phase, you add or subtract calories to get you back to a good maintenance phase-again doing this slowly so you can determine what the new set point is for yourself and avoid the "OMG I've gained 15 pounds in a week from adding in 1000 calories." If you haven't noticed, nutrition, like lifting, is highly individualized and may take a few adjustments to find that sweet spot that works for you.

**EATING DISORDERS:** Food for me has always been fuel and I never looked at anything as good, bad, or attached any emotion to it.  However, I do realize there are people that struggle with eating disorders and emotional attachments to food. In those cases it's really important to seek the help of a qualified nutritionist or therapist who has experience in this arena--it's ok to ask for help if you need it.

**MEAL PREP:** The better prepared you are, the easier it is. Meal prep is a necessary evil if you want to be successful. There are a lot of companies that will deliver to your door, however, if you're on a budget, this isn't the most economical. I think people really over complicate this part of dieting. Like I said earlier, my approach is to keep it simple. Therefore I tend to eat the same things for each meal during the week (minus dinner) when my schedule is busier and get more creative on the weekends when I have more time. Easy things to cook in bulk are rice (rice cooker), Ground turkey, beef, or chicken (cooks up really fast), and frozen veggies; convenient and keep longer than fresh ones. Need more help? Check out eatthismuch.com which will create a customized meal plans based on your caloric needs, budget and food likes--and it's free.

**WHAT ABOUT THE KIDS?** As a mom, I realize my kid's needs aren't on a diet. Therefore I think about meals that they'll also enjoy that won't require me to cook three different things. Most

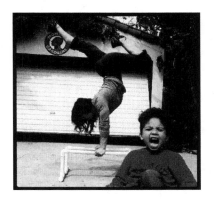

things can be made healthier and to fit your macros, but here are a few ideas that are easy to make multiple ways. Tacos, for instance, can be assembled (taco shells) or disassembled (taco salad) if you're out of carbs for the day. Spaghetti is another option that can be prepared for everyone to enjoy with or without pasta.

**SOCIAL SITUATIONS:** Unless you have no friends social situations that involve food can't and shouldn't be avoided. That being said, this is where you use common sense, the only caveat being if you're getting ready for a physique show, this will most likely mean you'll need to pack your food. However, show prep is only for a specified amount of time and that level of strictness isn't going to be the case for most of us. There is ALWAYS healthy options on the menu-if you choose to have that fried blooming onion as an appetizer though, try some portion control (share with your friends) and when you order your main meal opt for the veggies instead of the potato-since the deep fried onion was high in fat a good compromise is to cut out the starchy carb. This doesn't mean you failed, should feel guilty, and all is lost-it just means you get back on track for the next meal. Pretty simple right?

**PORTIONS AND PORTION CONTROL:** I'm a huge fan of not carrying around a scale to weigh your food forever. That's not real life and I think for general nutrition purposes everyone should learn what their portions look like. My typical protein portion is 3-4 oz--roughly the size of my palm. If you've measured your food for a while, you should be pretty good about knowing how much you should be consuming, especially because most of us eat the same things day in and day out. The best way to learn portion control that I've found, especially if eating in a restaurant, is portion out the food that fit your caloric needs and get the rest to go--once it's boxed up you're less likely to overeat and you have a meal for later. It takes practice, but once you get the hang of it, self control gets easier.

**BEING HUNGRY IS OK:** When you're in a cutting phase there are gonna be times when you're hungry-this is normal. You've reduced your calories and it takes some time to adjust. Sometimes this also means you're just not hydrated enough and drinking more water will solve the problem.

**STEPPING ON THE SCALE:** Stepping on the scale is really important to gauge weight gain or loss through the different dieting phases. However, stepping on the scale multiple times a day will serve no purpose and hinder your progress. Women experience weight fluctuations throughout the day so keep your weigh-ins to 2 times (for example Tuesday and Saturday at the same time)-this is sufficient to keep you accountable and determine if what you're doing is working without driving yourself crazy.

Your nutrition should match your training block and physique goals. To that end having a plan is crucial--if you're new to lifting plan on spending more time in a higher volume phase (this is the phase that adds muscle) and match your nutrition to that block. Higher volume phases are perfect for cutting or massing. If you're getting ready for a powerlifting meet and you're in the peaking phase that's the best time to be in maintenance mode-you want to be right around your competition weight when under the heavier loads-huge weight loss during this time can affect your lifts, especially the bench for women.

# PUTTING IT
# ALL TOGETHER

So now that you have all this information where do you start? I think most of us step foot into the gym to feel and look better. Therefore I would take a good look at your body Composition-where you currently are versus your desired look. Keep in mind the desired look may be a long term goal (remember it takes women longer to put on muscle) so plan accordingly and set short term realistic goals. If you want to get leaner or add muscle, you're gonna need to be doing more volume and the higher volume hypertrophy block is the best place to start. Determine how long you'll need to stay in this block to reach your desired goal and line up your nutrition to match--the volume in this block lends itself to either massing or cutting.

If you're planning on competing in powerlifting, you're going to need to know your competition schedule. The further away you are from your meet means you can spend more time in hypertrophy and strength blocks. Don't be alarmed that you're not always maxing out. These blocks are where you work on adding muscle, honing in good technique on the competition lifts, and increasing your work capacity. The more muscle you have, the stronger you will be on the platform--not to mention you decrease your risk of injury by not always putting your body under maximal loads. When I first started I did one to two meets max per year--even now the most I'll do is three and they are spread out pretty evenly to give me more time using lighter weight loads.

Finally, be consistent and don't stray from the plan. If you want to get leaner, add more muscle or be stronger, you have to be focused and see your plan through--this way you can determine what is working and what isn't. If you're constantly stopping and restarting or jumping from program to program you'll never know what changes need to be made to improve. Realize that this is a process, there will be ups, downs, frustrations as well as successes but there's no better feeling than following through. Seeing what your body is capable of and enjoying the journey to get it there is the most rewarding part.

# F.A.Q.
# WOMEN AND WEIGHT TRAINING

## WILL LIFTING MAKE ME BULKY / MANLY LOOKING?

This subject has been hammered to death, so I'll simply repeat what has been stated in blog post after blog post: women DO NOT have the same hormonal makeup as men, therefore putting on large amounts of muscle is not going to happen. Lifting will add muscle to your frame, but how "big" you look is also dependent on your bodyfat levels--the leaner you are, the more muscular and thus "bigger" you will appear. How you look is in YOUR control through training and nutrition.

## CAN I TRAIN WHILE PREGNANT?

Always consult your doctor before continuing an exercise program while pregnant. As long as there are no complications and you are healthy, training is actually good for you. By no means does this mean you get pregnant and decide training for a marathon is your next fitness goal. I'm talking about continuing with activities to which your body was already accustomed.  Listen to your doctor and your body, and above all be smart. Stay off your stomach and adapt exercises to your changing body. When you're seven months pregnant, lying hamstring curls aren't the best idea, let alone comfortable. I trained throughout both my pregnancies--doing so can make your labor easier and helps to keep some semblance of normalcy in your life, especially if you are used to being active and training heavy. You have to keep in mind that this is a time when you're not trying to add to your total, have a six pack, and set new records--training while pregnant is more about maintenance and preserving the muscle you already have.

When you are used to looking a certain way it is scary to see your body change, but let me assure you the body is amazing and with proper nutrition and continued activity you'll regain your pre-baby body.

## WILL MY UPPER BODY ALWAYS BE WEAK?

It's true that women tend to be weaker than men in this area, but stop saying it! If you say it enough, you eventually start believing it. The only way you overcome a weakness is to work at it. Women can handle more volume and frequency than men, so get after it and start working that upper body more often.

## AM I TOO OLD TO START?

You're never too old to start strength training. In fact, as we age we need to be stronger to be better in everyday activities. Not only does it help with confidence, but it helps with diseases like osteoporosis, diabetes, high blood pressure, and heart disease. It's one of the few activities that isn't exclusive to the twenty somethings--as a matter of fact in the IPF (International Powerlifting Federation) the top female athletes are all in their 40s.

# BEGINNER PROGRAM

As a beginner powerlifter it is important that you give yourself frequent exposure to the exercises. This is necessary because technique is lost quickly without practice, also because you are newer to the training, you won't have the ability to generate high levels of fatigue from training, so frequent training is needed to produce sufficient stimulus.

The Beginner's Program will take you through 4 Three-Week long blocks, giving you exposure to a variety of movement patterns to develop a broad base of strength and fitness while also developing your technique in the squat, bench and deadlift.

# BLOCK 1 / WEEK 1

| DAY 1: | DAY 2: | DAY 3: |
|---|---|---|
| 4" BLOCK PULL | BENCH PRESS | HI BAR SQUAT |
| 4x5 at 7RPE | Find a 10rm,Drop 12-15%x2x10 | 6x3 at 7RPE-1 min rests |
| DB INCLINE BENCH | FRONT FOOT ELEVATED | BARBELL PUSHUPS |
| 3x8-10 at 7RPE | SPLIT SQUATS | 3xFailure-3 min rest periods |
| GOBLET SQUAT | 3x6 each leg | DB RDLS |
| 4x8 at 8RPE | LAT PULLDOWNS | 3x8 at 7RPE |
| DB ROWS | 5x10-12 at 8RPE | CABLE ROWS |
| 4x10-12 at 8RPE | HAMSTRING CURLS | 3x10-12 at 8RPE |
| DB LATERAL RAISES | 3x12-15 at 7RPE | BACK RAISES |
| 3x8-10 | TRICEP PUSHDOWNS | 3x12 |
| | 3x15-20 at 8RPE | |

# BLOCK 1 / WEEK 2

| DAY 1: | DAY 2: | DAY 3: |
|---|---|---|
| 4" BLOCK PULL | BENCH PRESS | HI BAR SQUAT |
| 5x5 at 7RPE | Up to 10rm, Drop 12-15%x3x10 | 8x3 at 7RPE-1 min rest |
| DB INCLINE BENCH | FRONT FOOT ELEVATED | BARBELL PUSHUPS |
| 3x10-12 at 8RPE | SPLIT SQUATS | 3xFailure-3 min rest periods |
| GOBLET SQUAT | 3x8 each leg | DB RDLS |
| 4x8 at 8RPE | LAT PULLDOWNS | 3x10 at 7RPE |
| DB ROWS | 5x10-12 at 8RPE | CABLE ROWS |
| 4x10-12 at 8RPE | HAMSTRING CURLS | 3x10-12 at 8RPE |
| DB LATERAL RAISES | 3x12-15 at 7RPE | BACK RAISES |
| 3x10-12 | TRICEP PUSHDOWNS | 3x15 |
| | 3x15-20 at 8RPE | |

# BLOCK 1 / WEEK 3

| DAY 1: | DAY 2: | DAY 3: |
|---|---|---|
| 4" BLOCK PULL | BENCH PRESS | HI BAR SQUAT |
| 6x5 at 7RPE | Find a 10rm, Drop 12-15%x4x10 | 10x3 at 7RPE-1 min rest |
| DB INCLINE BENCH | FRONT FOOT ELEVATED | BARBELL PUSHUPS |
| 3x12-15 at 9RPE | SPLIT SQUATS | 3xFailure-3 min rest periods |
| GOBLET SQUAT | 3x10 each leg | DB RDLS |
| 4x12 at 8RPE | LAT PULLDOWNS | 3x12 at 7RPE |
| DB ROWS | 5x10-12 at 8RPE | CABLE ROWS |
| 4x10-12 at 8RPE | HAMSTRING CURLS | 3x10-12 at 8RPE |
| | 3x12-15 at 7RPE | BACK RAISES |
| | TRICEP PUSHDOWNS | 3x20 |
| | 3x15-20 at 8RPE | |

# BLOCK 2 / WEEK 1

### DAY 1:

4" BLOCK PULL
6x5 at 7RPE
DB INCLINE BENCH
3x12-15 at 9RPE
GOBLET SQUAT
4x12 at 8RPE
DB ROWS
4x10-12 at 8RPE

### DAY 2:

BENCH PRESS
Find an 8rm, Drop 8-12% 3x8
GOBLET SQUAT
3x10
REVERSE GRIP PULLDOWNS
5x10-12 at 8RPE
BB GLUTE BRIDGE
3x8 at 7RPE
DB SKULLCRUSHERS
3x8-10

### DAY 3:

LOW BAR SQUAT
5x5 at 7RPE
PALMS IN DB PUSHUPS
3x10-12
RDLS
3x8 at 7RPE
DB CHEST SUPPORTED ROWS
3x10-12 at 8RPE
GOOD MORNINGS
3x8 at 7RPE

# BLOCK 2 / WEEK 2

### DAY 1:

2" BLOCK PULL
5x3 at 8RPE
FLOOR PRESS
4x7 at 8RPE
FRONT SQUAT
3x6 at 8RPE
BARBELL ROWS
4x8 at 8RPE
DB FRONT RAISES
3x10-12

### DAY 2:

BENCH PRESS
Find an 8rm, Drop 8-12% 4x8
GOBLET SQUAT
3x12
REVERSE GRIP PULLDOWNS
5x10-12 at 8RPE
BB GLUTE BRIDGE
3x10 at 7RPE
DB SKULLCRUSHERS
3x10-12

### DAY 3:

LOW BAR SQUAT
4x5 at 8RPE
PALMS IN DB PUSHUPS
3x10-12
RDLS
3x10 at 7RPE
DB CHEST SUPPORTED ROWS
3x10-12 at 8RPE
GOOD MORNINGS
3x10 at 7RPE

# BLOCK 2 / WEEK 3

### DAY 1:

2" BLOCK PULL
4x3 at 9RPE
FLOOR PRESS
4x6 at 9RPE
FRONT SQUAT
3x5 at 9RPE
BARBELL ROWS
4x10 at 8RPE
DB FRONT RAISES
3x12-15

### DAY 2:

BENCH PRESS
Find an 8rm, Drop 8-12%5x8
GOBLET SQUAT
3x15
REVERSE GRIP PULLDOWNS
5x10-12 at 8RPE
BB GLUTE BRIDGE
3x12 at 7RPE
DB SKULLCRUSHERS
3x12-15

### DAY 3:

LOW BAR SQUAT
3x5 at 9RPE
PALMS IN DB PUSHUPS
3x15-20
RDLS
3x12 at 7RPE
DB CHEST SUPPORTED ROWS
3x10-12 at 8RPE
GOOD MORNINGS
3x12 at 7RPE

# BLOCK 3 / WEEK 1

### DAY 1:

SUMO DEADLIFT
4x4 at 8RPE
CLOSEGRIP BENCH
4x8 at 7RPE
PAUSE HI BAR SQUAT
3x6 at 7RPE
DB ROWS
4x8-10 at 7RPE
DELT TRIAD
3x8 each

### DAY 2:

BENCH PRESS
Up to 5rm, Drop 8-12%x4x5
PAUSE FRONT SQUAT
3x6 at 7RPE
LAT PULLDOWNS
5x10-12 at 8RPE
HAMSTRING CURLS
3x8-10 at 7RPE
PUSHDOWNS
3x10-12

### DAY 3:

HI BAR SQUAT
5x4 at 7RPE
DB INCLINE BENCH
3x8-10 at 8RPE
DEADLIFT
3x3 at 7RPE
CABLE ROWS
3x10-12 at 8RPE
BACK RAISES
3x10

# BLOCK 3 / WEEK 2

| DAY 1: | DAY 2: | DAY 3: |
|--------|--------|--------|
| SUMO DEADLIFT | BENCH PRESS | HI BAR SQUAT |
| 4x5 at 8RPE | Up to 5rm, Drop 8-12%x5x5 | 5x5 at 7RPE |
| CLOSEGRIP BENCH | PAUSE FRONT SQUAT | DB INCLINE BENCH |
| 4x10 at 7RPE | 3x8 at 7RPE | 3x10-12 at 8RPE |
| PAUSE HI BAR SQUAT | LAT PULLDOWNS | DEADLIFT |
| 3x8 at 7RPE | 5x10-12 at 8RPE | 3x4 at 7RPE |
| DB ROWS | HAMSTRING CURLS | CABLE ROWS |
| 4x10-12 at 7RPE | 3x10-12 at 7RPE | 3x10-12 at 8RPE |
| DELT TRIAD | PUSHDOWNS | BACK RAISES |
| 3x10 each | 3x12-15 | 3x12 |

# BLOCK 3 / WEEK 3

| DAY 1: | DAY 2: | DAY 3: |
|--------|--------|--------|
| SUMO DEADLIFT | BENCH PRESS | HI BAR SQUAT |
| 4x6 at 8RPE | Up to 5rm, Drop 8-12%x6x5 | 5x6 at 7RPE |
| CLOSEGRIP BENCH | PAUSE FRONT SQUAT | DB INCLINE BENCH |
| 4x12 at 7RPE | 3x10 at 7RPE | 3x12-15 at 8RPE |
| PAUSE HI BAR SQUAT | LAT PULLDOWNS | DEADLIFT |
| 3x10 at 7RPE | 5x10-12 at 8RPE | 3x5 at 7RPE |
| DB ROWS | HAMSTRING CURLS | CABLE ROWS |
| 4x12-15 at 7RPE | 3x10-15 at 7RPE | 3x10-12 at 8RPE |
| DELT TRIAD | PUSHDOWNS | BACK RAISES |
| 3x12 each | 3x15-20 | 3x15 |

# BLOCK 4 / WEEK 1

| DAY 1: | DAY 2: | DAY 3: |
|--------|--------|--------|
| DEADLIFT | BENCH PRESS | LOW BAR SQUAT |
| 5x3 at 7RPE | Up to 3rm, Drop 8-12%x4x3 | Up to 3rm at 8RPE, |
| WIDEGRIP BENCH | FRONT SQUAT | Drop 8-12%x3x3 |
| 4x6 at 7RPE | 3x5 at 8RPE | DB FLOOR PRESS |
| HI BAR SQUAT | REVERSE GRIP PULLDOWNS | 3x10 at 7RPE |
| 3x6 at 7RPE | 5x10-12 at 8RPE | SUMO DEADLIFT |
| BARBELL ROWS | BB GLUTE BRIDGE | 3x5 at 7RPE |
| 4x8 at 8RPE | 3x12 at 7RPE | DB CHEST SUPPORTED ROWS |
| SHOULDER BOX | DB SKULLCRUSHERS | 3x12 at 8RPE |
| 3x8 | 3x12 at 8RPE | GOOD MORNINGS |
|  |  | 3x12 at 7RPE |

# BLOCK 4 / WEEK 2

| DAY 1: | DAY 2: | DAY 3: |
|--------|--------|--------|
| DEADLIFT | BENCH PRESS | LOW BAR SQUAT |
| 4x3 at 8RPE | Up to 2rm, Drop 8-12%x3x2 | 5x3 at 7RPE |
| WIDEGRIP BENCH | FRONT SQUAT | DB FLOOR PRESS |
| 4x5 at 7-8RPE | 3x4 at 8RPE | 3x8 at 8RPE |
| HI BAR SQUAT | REVERSE GRIP PULLDOWNS | SUMO DEADLIFT |
| 3x5 at 7-8RPE | 5x10-12 at 8RPE | 3x4 at 7-8RPE |
| BARBELL ROWS | BB GLUTE BRIDGE | DB CHEST SUPPORTED ROWS |
| 4x6 at 8RPE | 3x10 at 7RPE | 3x10 at 8RPE |
| SHOULDER BOX | DB SKULLCRUSHERS | GOOD MORNINGS |
| 3x8 | 3x10 at 8RPE | 3x10 at 7RPE |

# BLOCK 4 / WEEK 3

## DAY 1:

DEADLIFT
Up to 3rm
WIDEGRIP BENCH
4x4 at 8RPE
HI BAR SQUAT
3x4 at 8RPE
BARBELL ROWS
4x5 at 8RPE
SHOULDER BOX
3x8

## DAY 2:

BENCH PRESS
Up to 1rm, Drop 8-12%x2x1
FRONT SQUAT
3x3 at 8RPE
REVERSE GRIP PULLDOWNS
5x10-12 at 8RPE
BB GLUTE BRIDGE
3x8 at 7RPE
DB SKULLCRUSHERS
3x8z at 8RPE

## DAY 3:

LOW BAR SQUAT
Up to 3rm at 10RPE,
Drop 8-12%x2x3
DB FLOOR PRESS
3x6 at 9RPE
SUMO DEADLIFT
3x3 at 8RPE
DB CHEST SUPPORTED ROWS
3x8 at 8RPE
GOOD MORNINGS
3x8 at 7RPE

# MOMSTRONG
# PROGRAM

MomStrong is a program designed to combine all elements of my training, Powerlifting, Bodybuilding, and Calisthenics into one fun and effective 12-week journey. This program will help you build muscle, hone your strength and technique in the powerlifts and maybe even get your first pullup.

# PHASE 1 / WEEK 1

## DAY 1:

HIGH BAR SQUAT
60%x3x8-10
HACK SQUAT, LEG PRESS
OR BELT SQUAT
3x10 at 8RPE
FRONT FOOT ELEVATED SPLIT SQUATS
3x10 at 8RPE
HAMSTRING CURLS OR GHR
3x10 at 8RPE
BACK RAISES
2x10 at 8RPE
CALF RAISES
3x15 at 8RPE

## DAY 2:

BENCH
70%x4x6-8
CLOSEGRIP BENCH
65%x3x6
INCLINE DB BENCH
3x10-12 at 8RPE
BETOVER ROWS
3x10-12 at 8RPE
LAT PULLDOWNS
3x12 at 8RPE
SEATED DB LATERAL RAISES
3x12 at 8RPE
FACE PULLS
3x12 at 8RPE
DEADHANG FROM PULLUP BAR
3x5-10 seconds

## DAY 3: CARDIO (20 mins)

## DAY 4:

CONVENTIONAL DEADLIFT
70%x3x6-8
3" SUMO BLOCK PULLS
65%x3x8
LOW BAR SQUAT
60%x3x8
BB HIP THRUSTS
3x10 at 8RPE
PULLTHROUGHS
3x10 at 8RPE
CALF RAISES
3x15 at 8RPE

## DAY 5:

WIDEGRIP BENCH
60%x4x8-10
DB INCLINE FLIES
3x12 at 8RPE
DB MILITARY PRESS
3x10 at 8RPE
DB FRONT RAISES
3x10 at 8RPE
TRICEP PUSHDOWNS
3x8-10
MILITARY PUSHUPS
3xAMRAP
INVERTED ROWS
3x10
PLANKS
3x30 sec

## DAY 6: CARDIO (20 mins)
## DAY 7: OFF

# PHASE 1 / WEEK 2

## DAY 1:

HIGH BAR SQUAT
70%x4x6
FRONT SQUAT
65%x3x8
SNATCH GRIP DEADLIFT
65%x3x8-10
HAMSTRING CURLS OR GHR
3x10 at 8RPE
CALF RAISES
3x15 at 8RPE

## DAY 2:

BENCH
60%x4x10
SPOTO PRESS
55%x3x8
DB ROWS
3x10 at 8RPE
PALMS IN DB PRESS
3x10-12 at 8RPE
DB LATERAL RAISES
3x10 at 8RPE
DB REVERSE FLIES
3x10 at 8RPE
SCAPULAR RETRACTIONS
FROM PULLUP BAR
3x6-8
HANGING LEG RAISES
3x15

## DAY 3: CARDIO (25 mins)

## DAY 4:

CONVENTIONAL DEADLIFT
60%x4x8
SUMO PAUSE DEADLIFTS
55%x3x8
LOW BAR SQUAT
65%X3X8
SETP UPS
3x8-10 each leg
SINGLE LEG GLUTE BRIDGES
3x12 each leg
CALF RAISES
3x15 at 8RPE

## DAY 5:

WIDEGRIP BENCH
70%x4x6
DB FLIES
3x10-12 at 8RPE
SINGLE ARM DB PRESS
3x10-12 at 8RPE
DB PULLOVERS
3x10 at 8RPE
DB SKULLCRUSHERS
3x10-12 at 8RPE
BAND ASSISTED OR
JUMPING PULLUPS
8, 8, 6
PLANKS
3x45 sec

## DAY 6: CARDIO (20 mins)
## DAY 7: OFF

# PHASE 1 / WEEK 3

## DAY 1:

HIGH BAR SQUAT
65%x4x8
HACK SQUAT, LEG PRESS
OR BELT SQUAT
3x10 at 8RPE
FRONT FOOT ELEVATED SPLIT SQUATS
3x10 at 8RPE
HAMSTRING CURLS OR GHR
3x10 at 8RPE
BACK RAISES
2x10 at 8RPE
CALF RAISES
3x15 at 8RPE

## DAY 2:

BENCH
75%x4x6
CLOSEGRIP BENCH
70%x3x6
INCLINE DB BENCH
3x10-12 at 8RPE
BETOVER ROWS
3x10-12 at 8RPE
LAT PULLDOWNS
3x12 at 8RPE
SEATED DB LATERAL RAISES
3x12 at 8RPE
FACE PULLS
3x12 at 8RPE
DEADHANG FROM PULLUP BAR
3x5-10 seconds

## DAY 3: CARDIO (30 mins)

## DAY 4:

CONVENTIONAL DEADLIFT
75%x4x6
3" SUMO BLOCK PULLS
70%x3x6
LOW BAR SQUAT
68%x3x8
BB HIP THRUSTS
3x10 at 8RPE
PULLTHROUGHS
3x10 at 8RPE
CALF RAISES
3x15 at 8RPE

## DAY 5:

WIDEGRIP BENCH
65%x4x8-10
DB INCLINE FLIES
3x12 at 8RPE
DB MILITARY PRESS
3x10 at 8RPE
DB FRONT RAISES
3x10 at 8RPE
TRICEP PUSHDOWNS
3x8-10
MILITARY PUSHUPS
3xAMRAP
INVERTED ROWS
4x10
PLANKS
3x60 sec

## DAY 6: CARDIO (30 mins)
## DAY 7: OFF

# PHASE 1 / WEEK 4

## DAY 1:

HIGH BAR SQUAT
75%x4x6
FRONT SQUAT
70%x3x6
SNATCH GRIP DEADLIFT
70%x3x8
HAMSTRING CURLS OR GHR
3x10 at 8RPE
CALF RAISES
3x15 at 8RPE

## DAY 2:

BENCH
65%x4x8-10
SPOTO PRESS
60%x3x8
DB ROWS
3x10 at 8RPE
PALMS IN DB PRESS
3x10-12 at 8RPE
DB LATERAL RAISES
3x10 at 8RPE
DB REVERSE FLIES
3x10 at 8RPE
SCAPULAR RETRACTIONS
FROM PULLUP BAR
3x6-8
HANGING LEG RAISES
3x15

## DAY 3: CARDIO (30 mins)

## DAY 4:

CONVENTIONAL DEADLIFT
65%x4x8
SUMO PAUSE DEADLIFTS
60%x3x8
LOW BAR SQUAT
70%x3x6
SETP UPS
3x8-10 each leg
SINGLE LEG GLUTE BRIDGES
3x12 each leg
CALF RAISES
3x15 at 8RPE

## DAY 5:

WIDEGRIP BENCH
75%x4x6
DB FLIES
3x10-12 at 8RPE
SINGLE ARM DB PRESS
3x10-12 at 8RPE
DB PULLOVERS
3x10 at 8RPE
DB SKULLCRUSHERS
3x10-12 at 8RPE
BAND ASSISTED OR
JUMPING PULLUPS
10, 8, 6
PLANKS
3x60 sec

## DAY 6: CARDIO (30 mins)
## DAY 7: OFF

# PHASE 1 / WEEK 5

## DAY 1:

HIGH BAR SQUAT
70%x4x8
HACK SQUAT, LEG PRESS
OR BELT SQUAT
3x10 at 8RPE
FRONT FOOT ELEVATED SPLIT SQUATS
3x10 at 8RPE
HAMSTRING CURLS OR GHR
3x10 at 8RPE
BACK RAISES
2x10 at 8RPE
CALF RAISES
3x15 at 8RPE

## DAY 2:

BENCH
80%x4x6
CLOSEGRIP BENCH
75%x3x6
INCLINE DB BENCH
3x10-12 at 8RPE
BETOVER ROWS
3x10-12 at 8RPE
LAT PULLDOWNS
3x12 at 8RPE
SEATED DB LATERAL RAISES
3x12 at 8RPE
FACE PULLS
3x12 at 8RPE
DEADHANG FROM PULLUP BAR
3x5-10 seconds

## DAY 3: CARDIO (30 mins)

## DAY 4:

CONVENTIONAL DEADLIFT
80%x4x6
3" SUMO BLOCK PULLS
75%x3x6
LOW BAR SQUAT
73%x3x8
BB HIP THRUSTS
3x10 at 8RPE
PULLTHROUGHS
3x10 at 8RPE
CALF RAISES
3x15 at 8RPE

## DAY 5:

WIDEGRIP BENCH
70%x4x8
DB INCLINE FLIES
3x12 at 8RPE
DB MILITARY PRESS
3x10 at 8RPE
DB FRONT RAISES
3x10 at 8RPE
TRICEP PUSHDOWNS
3x8-10
MILITARY PUSHUPS
3xAMRAP
INVERTED ROWS
3x12
PLANKS
3x60 sec

## DAY 6: CARDIO (30 mins)
## DAY 7: OFF

# PHASE 1 / WEEK 6

## DAY 1:

HIGH BAR SQUAT
80%x4x6
FRONT SQUAT
73%x3x6
SNATCH GRIP DEADLIFT
73%x3x6
HAMSTRING CURLS OR GHR
3x10 at 8RPE
CALF RAISES
3x15 at 8RPE

## DAY 2:

BENCH
70%x4x8
SPOTO PRESS
63%x3x8
DB ROWS
3x10 at 8RPE
PALMS IN DB PRESS
3x10-12 at 8RPE
DB LATERAL RAISES
3x10 at 8RPE
DB REVERSE FLIES
3x10 at 8RPE
SCAPULAR RETRACTIONS
FROM PULLUP BAR
3x6-8
HANGING LEG RAISES
3x15

## DAY 3: CARDIO (30 mins)

## DAY 4:

CONVENTIONAL DEADLIFT
70%x4x8
SUMO PAUSE DEADLIFTS
65%x3x8
LOW BAR SQUAT
75%x3x5
SETP UPS
3x8-10 each leg
SINGLE LEG GLUTE BRIDGES
3x12 each leg
CALF RAISES
3x15 at 8RPE

## DAY 5:

WIDEGRIP BENCH
80%x4x6
DB FLIES
3x10-12 at 8RPE
SINGLE ARM DB PRESS
3x10-12 at 8RPE
DB PULLOVERS
3x10 at 8RPE
DB SKULLCRUSHERS
3x10-12 at 8RPE
BAND ASSISTED OR
JUMPING PULLUPS
10, 10, 8
PLANKS
3x60 sec

## DAY 6: CARDIO (30 mins)
## DAY 7: OFF

# PHASE 2 / WEEK 1

## DAY 1:

LOW BAR SQUAT
65%x3x6
HACK SQUAT, LEG PRESS
OR BELT SQUAT
2x10 at 8RPE
FRONT FOOT ELEVATED SPLIT SQUATS
2x10 at 8RPE
HAMSTRING CURLS OR GHR
2x10 at 8RPE
BACK RAISES
2x10 at 8RPE
CALF RAISES
3x15 at 8RPE

## DAY 2:

BENCH
65%x3x6
PALMS IN DB PRESS
2x10 at 8RPE
LAT PULLDOWNS
3x10 at 8RPE
FACE PULLS
2x10 at 8RPE
SEATED DB LATERAL RAISES
2x10 at 8RPE
DEADHANG FROM PULLUP BAR
2x5-10 sec
HANGING LEG RAISES
3x15

## DAY 3: CARDIO (30 mins)

## DAY 4:

CONVENTIONAL DEADLIFT
70%x3x6
HIGH BAR SQUAT
60%x3x6
BB HIP THRUSTS
2x10 at 8RPE
PULLTHROUGHS
2x10 at 8RPE
CALF RAISES
3x15 at 8RPE

## DAY 5:

DB INCLINE BENCH
3x10 at 8RPE
DB MILITARY PRESS
3x10 at 8RPE
DB FRONT RAISES
2x10 at 8RPE
DB REVERSE FLIES
2x10 at 8RPE
INVERTED ROWS
3x10
PLANKS
3x1 min

## DAY 6: CARDIO (30 mins)
## DAY 7: OFF

# PHASE 2 / WEEK 2

## DAY 1:

LOW BAR SQUAT
85%x2x3, 75%x2x4
PAUSE BELOW PARALLEL SQUAT
70%x2x5
HACK SQUAT, LEG PRESS
OR BELT SQUAT
2x10 at 8RPE
HAMSTRING CURLS OR GHR
2x10 at 8RPE
CALF RAISES
3x15 at 8RPE

## DAY 2:

BENCH
75%x4x6
SPOTO PRESS
70%x3x6
DB ROWS
3x10 at 8RPE
DB LATERAL RAISES
3x10-12 at 8RPE
DB REVERSE FLIES
3x10 at 8RPE
PARTIAL PULLUPS
(as big ROM as you can)
4x2
HANGING LEG RAISES
3x15

## DAY 3: CARDIO (25 mins)

## DAY 4:

CONVENTIONAL DEADLIFT
75%x4x5
1" DEFICIT DEADLIFT
70%x3x5
HIGH BAR SQUAT
70%x3x5
BACK RAISES
2x10 at 8RPE
CALF RAISES
3x15 at 8RPE

## DAY 5:

WIDEGRIP BENCH
80%x2x8, 70%x2x5
DB INCLINE BENCH
3x10 at 8RPE
SINGLE ARM DB PRESS
3x10-12 at 8RPE
DB PULLOVERS
3x10 at 8RPE
DB SKULLCRUSHERS
3x10-12 at 8RPE
INVERTED ROWS
3x10
PLANKS
3x1 min

## DAY 6: CARDIO (25 mins)
## DAY 7: OFF

# PHASE 2 / WEEK 3

## DAY 1:

LOW BAR SQUAT
75%x4x5
PAUSE ABOVE PARALLEL SQUAT
70%x3x5
HACK SQUAT, LEG PRESS
OR BELT SQUAT
3x10 at 8RPE
HAMSTRING CURLS OR GHR
2x10 at 8RPE
CALF RAISES
3x15 at 8RPE

## DAY 2:

BENCH
85%x2x3, 75%x2x5
CLOSEGRIP BENCH
73%x2x5
INCLINE DB BENCH
2x10 at 8RPE
BENTOVER ROWS
3x10 at 8RPE
LAT PULLDOWNS
2x10 at 8RPE
SEATED DB LATERAL RAISES
2x10 at 8RPE
FACE PULLS
2x10 at 8RPE
INVERTED ROWS
2x10 at 8RPE

## DAY 3: CARDIO (30 mins)

## DAY 4:

CONVENTIONAL DEADLIFT
85%x3, 75%x2x4
3" CONVENTIONAL BLOCK PULLS
70%x3x3
HIGH BAR SQUAT
73%x3x5
BACK RAISES
2x10 at 8RPE
CALF RAISES
3x15 at 8RPE

## DAY 5:

WIDEGRIP BENCH
75%x3x6
DB INCLINE BENCH
3x10 at 8RPE
DB MILITARY PRESS
3x10 at 8RPE
DB FRONT RAISES
3x10 at 8RPE
TRICEP PUSHDOWNS
3x10 at 8RPE
PARTIAL PULLUPS
5x2
PLANKS
3x1 min

## DAY 6: CARDIO (30 mins)
## DAY 7: OFF

# PHASE 2 / WEEK 4

## DAY 1:

LOW BAR SQUAT
90%x2, 80%x2x3
PAUSE BELOW PARALLEL SQUAT
75%x2x4
HAMSTRING CURLS OR GHR
2x10 at 8RPE
CALF RAISES
3x15 at 8RPE

## DAY 2:

BENCH
80%x4x3
SPOTO PRESS
75%x3x5
DB ROWS
3x10 at 8RPE
PALMS IN DB BENCH
2x10 at 8RPE
DB LATERAL RAISES
2x10 at 8RPE
DB REVERSE FLIES
2x10 at 8RPE
PARTIAL PULLUPS
5x3
HANGING LEG RAISES
3x15

## DAY 3: CARDIO (30 mins)

## DAY 4:

CONVENTIONAL DEADLIFT
80%x5x1
1" DEFICIT DEADLIFT
75%x2x4
HIGH BAR SQUAT
75%x3x5
BACK RAISES
2x10 at 8RPE
CALF RAISES
3x15 at 8RPE

## DAY 5:

WIDEGRIP BENCH
78%x3x5
DB INCLINE BENCH
3x8 at 8RPE
SINGLE ARM DB PRESS
2x10 at 8RPE
DB PULLOVERS
2x10 at 8RPE
DB SKULLCRUSHERS
2x10-12 at 8RPE
INVERTED ROWS
2x10
PLANKS
3x1 min

## DAY 6: CARDIO (30 mins)
## DAY 7: OFF

# PHASE 2 / WEEK 5

## DAY 1:

LOW BAR SQUAT
80%x4x3
PAUSE ABOVE PARALLEL SQUAT
75%x2x4
HACK SQUAT, LEG PRESS
OR BELT SQUAT
2x10 at 8RPE
HAMSTRING CURLS OR GHR
2x10 at 8RPE
CALF RAISES
3x15 at 8RPE

## DAY 2:

BENCH
Up to 1rm, Drop 10-15%x3x4
BENTOVER ROWS
2x10 at 8RPE
LAT PULLDOWNS
2x10 at 8RPE
SEATED DB LATERAL RAISES
2x10 at 8RPE
FACE PULLS
2x10 at 8RPE
INVERTED ROWS
3x10

## DAY 3: CARDIO (30 mins)

## DAY 4:

CONVENTIONAL DEADLIFT
Up to 1rm
HACK SQUAT, LEG PRESS
OR BELT SQUAT
2x10 at 8RPE
HIGH BAR SQUAT
78%x3x3
BACK RAISES
2x10 at 8RPE
CALF RAISES
3x15 at 8RPE

## DAY 5:

INCLINE DB BENCH
3x10 at 8RPE
DB INCLINE FLIES
3x10 at 8RPE
DB MILITARY PRESS
3x10 at 8RPE
DB FRONT RAISES
3x10 at 8RPE
DB SKULLCRUSHERS
2x10 at 8RPE
DIPS
2x10
PARTIAL PULLUPS
6x3
PLANKS
3x1 min

## DAY 6: CARDIO (30 mins)
## DAY 7: OFF

# PHASE 2 / WEEK 6

## DAY 1:

LOW BAR SQUAT
Up to 1rm
HACK SQUAT, LEG PRESS
OR BELT SQUAT
2x10 at 8RPE
HAMSTRING CURLS OR GHR
2x10 at 8RPE
CALF RAISES
3x15 at 8RPE

## DAY 2:

INCLINE BENCH
3x10 at 8RPE
PUSHUPS
4x10
DB ROWS
3x10 at 8RPE
DB LATERAL RAISES
3x10 at 8RPE
DB REVERSE FLIES
3x10 at 8RPE
TRICEP PUSHDOWNS
3x10 at 8RPE
INVERTED ROWS
3x10
HANGING LEG RAISES
3x15

## DAY 3: CARDIO (OFF)

## DAY 4:

SUMO 3" BLOCK PULL
75%x3x5
HACK SQUAT, LEG PRESS
OR BELT SQUAT
3x10 at 8RPE
RDL
3x10 at 8RPE
PULLTHROUGHS
2x10 at 8RPE
CALF RAISES
3x15 at RPE

## DAY 5:

INCLINE DB BENCH
3x10 at 8RPE
DB INCLINE FLIES
3x10 at 8RPE
DB MILITARY PRESS
3x10 at 8RPE
DB FRONT RAISES
3x10 at 8RPE
DB SKULLCRUSHERS
2x10 at 8RPE
DIPS
2x10
PULLUPS
Max Reps
PLANKS
3x1 min

## DAY 6: CARDIO (OFF)
## DAY 7: OFF

# POWERLIFTING PROGRAM

This 5 Day/Week Powerlifting Program will progress you through three phases of training, Hypertrophy, Strength, and Peaking, applying the principles discussed in the Programming Considerations section of this book. Each phase has a specific goal, Hypertrophy is aimed at building muscle, Strength is geared towards improving force production and finally, Peaking will hone your technique and the skills of the 1 rep max.

# HYPERTROPHY BLOCK
## WEEK 1

### DAY 1

HIGH BAR SQUAT
Up to 10rm at 8RPE
HIGH BAR SQUAT
Drop 8-12%x2x10
FRONT SQUAT
2x8 at 7RPE
SPLIT SQUATS
2x8 each leg
BACK RAISES
3x10

### DAY 2

WIDEGRIP BENCH
Up to 10rm at 8RPE
WIDEGRIP BENCH
Drop 8-12%x3x10
DB INCLINE BENCH
3x8 at 7RPE
LAT PULLDOWNS
4x8-10, 1xCluster
DELT TRIAD
2-3x8 each
DB SKULLCRUSHERS
2x8, 1xRest Pause
DB CURLS
2-3x8

### DAY 3

CONVENTIONAL DEADLIFT
Up to 8rm at 8RPE
CONVENTIONAL DEADLIFT
Drop 8-12%x2x8
SNATCH GRIP RDL
3x6 at 7RPE
BELT SQUAT
2x10 at 7RPE
GLUTE BRIDGES
3x10
GHR
3x10

### DAY 4

OFF

### DAY 5

HIGH BAR 1-1/2 REP SQUATS
3x8 at 7RPE
LEG PRESS OR BELT SQUAT
2x10 at 7RPE
BOX DEADLIFT
2x8 at 7RPE
WALKING LUNGES
2x8 each leg
BACK RAISES
3x10

### DAY 6

INCLINE BENCH
3x8 at 7RPE
DB BENCH
3x8 at 7RPE
DB ROWS
4x8-10
DB FLIES
2-3x8
TRICEP PUSHDOWNS
2x8, 1xRest Pause
DB SHRUGS
2-3x8

# HYPERTROPHY BLOCK
# WEEK 2

| DAY 1 | DAY 2 | DAY 3 |
|-------|-------|-------|
| HIGH BAR SQUAT | WIDEGRIP BENCH | CONVENTIONAL DEADLIFT |
| Up to 10rm at 9RPE | Up to 10rm at 9RPE | 3" Blocks-85% of 8rm 2x8, 1xAMAP |
| HIGH BAR SQUAT | WIDEGRIP BENCH | CONVENTIONAL DEADLIFT |
| Drop 8-12%x3x10 | Drop 8-12%x4x10 | |
| FRONT SQUAT | DB INCLINE BENCH | SNATCH GRIP RDL |
| 2x8 at 8RPE | 3x10 at 8RPE | 3x8 at 8RPE |
| SPLIT SQUATS | LAT PULLDOWNS | BELT SQUAT |
| 2x10 each leg | 4x10-12, 1xCluster | 2x10 at 8RPE |
| BACK RAISES | DELT TRIAD | GLUTE BRIDGES |
| 3x12 | 2-3x10 each | 3x12 |
| | DB SKULLCRUSHERS | GHR |
| | 2x10, 1xRest Pause | 3x12 |
| | DB CURLS | |
| | 2-3x10 | |

| DAY 4 | DAY 5 | DAY 6 |
|-------|-------|-------|
| OFF | HIGH BAR 1-1/2 REP SQUATS | INCLINE BENCH |
| | 4x8 at 8RPE | 4x8 at 8RPE |
| | LEG PRESS OR BELT SQUAT | DB BENCH |
| | 2x10 at 8RPE | 3x10 at 8RPE |
| | BOX DEADLIFT | DB ROWS |
| | 2x8 at 8RPE | 4x10-12 |
| | WALKING LUNGES | DB FLIES |
| | 2x10 each leg | 2-3x10 |
| | BACK RAISES | TRICEP PUSHDOWNS |
| | 3x12 | 2x10, 1xRest Pause |
| | | DB SHRUGS |
| | | 2-3x10 |

# HYPERTROPHY BLOCK
# WEEK 3

## DAY 1

**HIGH BAR SQUAT**
Up to 10rm at 10RPE
**HIGH BAR SQUAT**
Drop 8-12%x4x10
**FRONT SQUAT**
2x8 at 9RPE
**SPLIT SQUATS**
2x12 each leg
**BACK RAISES**
3x15

## DAY 2

**WIDEGRIP BENCH**
Up to 10rm at 10RPE
**WIDEGRIP BENCH**
Drop 8-12%x5x10
**DB INCLINE BENCH**
3x12 at 9RPE
**LAT PULLDOWNS**
4x12-15, 1xCluster
**DELT TRIAD**
2-3x12 each
**DB SKULLCRUSHERS**
2x12, 1xRest Pause
**DB CURLS**
2-3x12

## DAY 3

**CONVENTIONAL DEADLIFT**
Up to 8rm at 10RPE
**CONVENTIONAL DEADLIFT**
Drop 8-12%x3x8
**SNATCH GRIP RDL**
3x10 at 9RPE
**BELT SQUAT**
2x10 at 9RPE
**GLUTE BRIDGES**
3x15
**GHR**
3x15

## DAY 4

OFF

## DAY 5

**HIGH BAR 1-1/2 REP SQUATS**
4x8 at 9RPE
**LEG PRESS OR BELT SQUAT**
2x10 at 9RPE
**BOX DEADLIFT**
2x8 at 9RPE
**WALKING LUNGES**
2x12 each leg
**BACK RAISES**
3x15

## DAY 6

**INCLINE BENCH**
4x8 at 9RPE
**DB BENCH**
3x12 at 9RPE
**DB ROWS**
4x12-15
**DB FLIES**
2-3x12
**TRICEP PUSHDOWNS**
2x12, 1xRest Pause
**DB SHRUGS**
2-3x12

# HYPERTROPHY BLOCK
# DELOAD

## DAY 1

HIGH BAR SQUAT
3x10 at 75% of 10rm
HIGH BAR SQUAT

FRONT SQUAT
2x6 at 7RPE
SPLIT SQUATS
2x8 each leg
BACK RAISES
3x10

## DAY 2

WIDEGRIP BENCH
4x10 at 75% of 10rm
WIDEGRIP BENCH

DB INCLINE BENCH
3x8 at 7RPE
LAT PULLDOWNS
4x8-12
DELT TRIAD
2x8 each
DB SKULLCRUSHERS
2x8
DB CURLS
2x8

## DAY 3

CONVENTIONAL DEADLIFT
2x8 at 75% of 8rm
CONVENTIONAL DEADLIFT

SNATCH GRIP RDL
3x6 at 7RPE
BELT SQUAT
2x8 at 7RPE
GLUTE BRIDGES
2x10
GHR
2x10

## DAY 4

OFF

## DAY 5

HIGH BAR 1-1/2 REP SQUATS
3x8 at 7RPE
LEG PRESS OR BELT SQUAT
2x8 at 7RPE
BOX DEADLIFT
2x8 at 7RPE
WALKING LUNGES
2x8 each leg
BACK RAISES
3x10

## DAY 6

INCLINE BENCH
3x8 at 7RPE
DB BENCH
2x8 at 7RPE
DB ROWS
4x8-12
DB FLIES
2x8
TRICEP PUSHDOWNS
2x8
DB SHRUGS
2x8

# STRENGTH BLOCK
# WEEK 1

## DAY 1

SQUAT
Up to 5rm at 8RPE
SQUAT
Drop 8-12%x4x5
PAUSE SQUAT
2x6 at 7RPE
STEP UPS
2x8 each leg
BACK RAISES
3x10

## DAY 2

BENCH
Up to 5rm at 8RPE
BENCH
Drop 8-12%x5x5
SPOTO PRESS
2x6 at 7RPE
LAT PULLDOWNS
4x8-10
DB FRONT RAISES
2-3x8
DB SKULLCRUSHERS
2-3x8
DB CURLS
2-3x8

## DAY 3

DEADLIFT
Up to 3rm at 8RPE
DEADLIFT
Drop 8-12%x3x3
BOX DEADLIFT
4x5 at 7RPE
GLUTE BRIDGES
3x10
GHR
3x10

## DAY 4

OFF

## DAY 5

HIGH BAR SQUATS
4x6 at 70-75%
LEG PRESS OR BELT SQUAT
3x8 at 7RPE
DEADLIFT
65-70%x3x5
SPLIT SQUATS
2x6 each leg
BACK RAISES
3x10

## DAY 6

INCLINE BENCH
3x6 at 7RPE
CLOSEGRIP BENCH
3x6 at 70-75%
DB ROWS
4x8-10
DB FLIES
2-3x8
TRICEP PUSHDOWNS
2-3x8
DB SHRUGS
2-3x8

# STRENGTH BLOCK
# WEEK 2

## DAY 1

SQUAT
Up to 4rm at 9RPE
SQUAT
Drop 8-12%x3x4
PAUSE SQUAT
2x5 at 7-8RPE
STEP UPS
2x8 each leg
BACK RAISES
3x10

## DAY 2

BENCH
Up to 4rm at 9RPE
BENCH
Drop 8-12%x4x4
SPOTO PRESS
2x5 at 7-8RPE
LAT PULLDOWNS
4x8-10
DB FRONT RAISES
2-3x8
DB SKULLCRUSHERS
2-3x8
DB CURLS
2-3x8

## DAY 3

DEADLIFT
3" Blocks: 4-5x3 at 8RPE
DEADLIFT

BOX DEADLIFT
4x5 at 7-8RPE
GLUTE BRIDGES
3x10
GHR
3x10

## DAY 4

OFF

## DAY 5

HIGH BAR SQUATS
4x5 at 72.5-77.5%
LEG PRESS OR BELT SQUAT
3x8 at 7-8RPE
DEADLIFT
70-75%x3x4
SPLIT SQUATS
2x6 each leg
BACK RAISES
3x10

## DAY 6

INCLINE BENCH
3x5 at 7-8RPE
CLOSEGRIP BENCH
3x5 at 75-80%
DB ROWS
4x8-10
DB FLIES
2-3x8
TRICEP PUSHDOWNS
2-3x8
DB SHRUGS
2-3x8

# STRENGTH BLOCK
# WEEK 3

## DAY 1

SQUAT
Up to 3rm at 10RPE
SQUAT
Drop 8-12%x2x3
PAUSE SQUAT
2x4 at 8RPE
STEP UPS
2x8 each leg
BACK RAISES
3x10

## DAY 2

BENCH
Up to 3rm at 10RPE
BENCH
Drop 8-12%x3x3
SPOTO PRESS
2x4 at 8RPE
LAT PULLDOWNS
4x8-10
DB FRONT RAISES
2-3x8
DB SKULLCRUSHERS
2-3x8
DB CURLS
2-3x8

## DAY 3

DEADLIFT
Up to 3rm at 10RPE
DEADLIFT
Drop 8-12%x2x3
BOX DEADLIFT
4x5 at 8RPE
GLUTE BRIDGES
3x10
GHR
3x10

## DAY 4

OFF

## DAY 5

HIGH BAR SQUATS
4x4 at 75-80%
LEG PRESS OR BELT SQUAT
3x8 at 8RPE
DEADLIFT
75-80%x3x3
SPLIT SQUATS
2x6 each leg
BACK RAISES
3x10

## DAY 6

INCLINE BENCH
3x4 at 8RPE
CLOSEGRIP BENCH
3x4 at 80-85%
DB ROWS
4x8-10
DB FLIES
2-3x8
TRICEP PUSHDOWNS
2-3x8
DB SHRUGS
2-3x8

# STRENGTH BLOCK
# DELOAD

## DAY 1

SQUAT
3x3 at 80% of 3rm
SQUAT

PAUSE SQUAT
2x4 at 6RPE
STEP UPS
2x8 each leg
BACK RAISES
2x10

## DAY 2

BENCH
3x3 at 80% of 3rm
BENCH

SPOTO PRESS
2x4 at 6RPE
LAT PULLDOWNS
3x8-10
DB FRONT RAISES
2x8
DB SKULLCRUSHERS
2x8
DB CURLS
2x8

## DAY 3

DEADLIFT
3x3 at 75% of 3rm
DEADLIFT

BOX DEADLIFT
3x5 at 6RPE
GLUTE BRIDGES
2x10
GHR
2x10

## DAY 4

OFF

## DAY 5

HIGH BAR SQUATS
3x4 at 70-75%
LEG PRESS OR BELT SQUAT
3x8 at 7RPE
DEADLIFT
70-75%x2x3
SPLIT SQUATS
2x6 each leg
BACK RAISES
2x10

## DAY 6

INCLINE BENCH
2x4 at 7RPE
CLOSEGRIP BENCH
2x4 at 70-75%
DB ROWS
3x8-10
DB FLIES
2x8
TRICEP PUSHDOWNS
2x8
DB SHRUGS
2x8

# PEAKING BLOCK
# WEEK 1

| DAY 1 | DAY 2 | DAY 3 |
|-------|-------|-------|
| DEADLIFT | OFF | BENCH |
| Up to 2rm at 8.5RPE | | Up to 2rm at 9.5RPE |
| DEADLIFT | | BENCH |
| Drop 6-10%x3x1 | | Drop 8-12%x3x2 |
| SQUAT | | SQUAT |
| 3x1 at 75-85%, 3x2 at 7080% | | 3x1 at 75-85%, 2x3 at 65-75% |
| BENCH | | LAT PULLDOWNS |
| 3x1 at 80-90%, 3x3 at 75-85% | | 5x6-10 |
| BOX DEADLIFT | | DB FRONT RAISES |
| 3x5 at 7-8RPE | | 2-3x8-12 |
| BACK RAISES | | DB SKULLCRUSHERS |
| 3x8-12 | | 2-3x8-12 |
| | | DB SHRUGS |
| | | 2-3x8-12 |

| DAY 4 | DAY 5 | DAY 6 |
|-------|-------|-------|
| OFF | SQUAT | WIDEGRIP BENCH |
| | Up to 2rm at 9RPE | 75%x3x5 |
| | SQUAT | CLOSEGRIP BENCH |
| | Drop 8-12%x2x2 | 75%x3x5 |
| | DEADLIFT | DB ROWS |
| | 3-5x1 at 70% | 4x6-10 |
| | GHR | DB FLIES |
| | 3x8-12 | 2x8-12 |
| | | DB LATERAL RAISES |
| | | 2x8-12 |
| | | TRICEP PUSHDOWNS |
| | | 2x8-12 |

# PEAKING BLOCK
# WEEK 2

| DAY 1 | DAY 2 | DAY 3 |
|---|---|---|

**DAY 1**

DEADLIFT
70%x9x1
DEADLIFT

SQUAT
3x1 at 77.5-87.5%, 2x2 at 75-82.5%
BENCH
3x1 at 82.5-92.5%, 2x3 at 77.5-85%
BOX DEADLIFT
3x4 at 8RPE
BACK RAISES
3x8-12

**DAY 2**

OFF

**DAY 3**

BENCH
4-6x3 at 80-85%
BENCH

SQUAT
3x1 at 77.5-87.5%, 1x3 at 67.5-77.5%
LAT PULLDOWNS
5x6-10
DB FRONT RAISES
2-3x8-12
DB SKULLCRUSHERS
2-3x8-12
DB SHRUGS
2-3x8-12

| DAY 4 | DAY 5 | DAY 6 |
|---|---|---|

**DAY 4**

OFF

**DAY 5**

SQUAT
3-5x3 at 77.5-85%
SQUAT

DEADLIFT
3-5x1 at 72.5%
GHR
3x8-12

**DAY 6**

WIDEGRIP BENCH
80%x3x4
CLOSEGRIP BENCH
80%x3x4
DB ROWS
4x6-10
DB FLIES
2x8-12
DB LATERAL RAISES
2x8-12
TRICEP PUSHDOWNS
2x8-12

# PEAKING BLOCK
# WEEK 3

| DAY 1 | DAY 2 | DAY 3 |
|---|---|---|
| DEADLIFT | OFF | BENCH |
| Up to 1rm at 9.5RPE | | Up to 1rm at 9.5RPE |
| DEADLIFT | | BENCH |
| Drop 6-10%x2x1 | | Drop 8-12%x2-3x1-2 |
| SQUAT | | SQUAT |
| 3x1 at 80-85%, 1x2 at 77.5-85% | | 3x1 at 80-90%, 1x3 at 70-80% |
| BENCH | | LAT PULLDOWNS |
| 3x1 at 85-95%, 1x3 at 80-87.5% | | 5x6-10 |
| BOX DEADLIFT | | DB FRONT RAISES |
| 3x3 at 8-9RPE | | 2-3x8-12 |
| BACK RAISES | | DB SKULLCRUSHERS |
| 3x8-12 | | 2-3x8-12 |
| | | DB SHRUGS |
| | | 2-3x8-12 |

| DAY 4 | DAY 5 | DAY 6 |
|---|---|---|
| OFF | SQUAT | WIDEGRIP BENCH |
| | Up to 1rm at 9.5RPE | 85%x3x3 |
| | SQUAT | CLOSEGRIP BENCH |
| | Drop 8-12%x2x1 | 85%x3x3 |
| | DEADLIFT | DB ROWS |
| | 3-5x1 at 75% | 4x6-10 |
| | GHR | DB FLIES |
| | 3x8-12 | 2x8-12 |
| | | DB LATERAL RAISES |
| | | 2x8-12 |
| | | TRICEP PUSHDOWNS |
| | | 2x8-12 |

# PEAKING BLOCK
# TAPER WEEK

| DAY 1 | DAY 2 | DAY 3 |
|---|---|---|
| DEADLIFT | OFF | BENCH |
| 65%x3-5x1 | | 70%x3-5x1, 60%x3 |
| SQUAT | | SQUAT |
| 75%x3-5x1, 65%x5 | | 65%x3-5x1, 55%x3 |
| BENCH | | DEADLIFT |
| 80%x3-5x1, 70%x5 | | 50%x3-5x1 |

| DAY 4 | DAY 5 | DAY 6 |
|---|---|---|
| OFF | LIGHT WARMUP | COMPETE |

# WORLD RECORD PROGRAM

This is the exact program Marisa used to train for the 2017 Arnold IPF Grand Prix. Marisa began this program with PRs of Squat: 145kg/319#, Bench: 90kg/198# and Deadlift: 182.5kg/402#, these are what we based the %s off of. The results of the training were Squat: 150kg/330#, Bench: 92.5kg/204#, Deadlift: 187.5kg/413# and the All-Time Total World Record.

This is program will take you through a four-week Hypertrophy Block + 1-week Deload, then a four week General Strength Block + 1-week Deload and finally finishing with a three week Peak and 1-week taper into competition.

# HYPERTROPHY BLOCK
# WEEK 1

## MONDAY

HIGH BAR SQUAT
65-70%x4x8
FRONT SQUAT
70-75%x3x8
SPLIT SQUAT
2x10 each leg
HAMSTRING CURLS
3x10

## TUESDAY

WIDEGRIP BENCH
70-75%x6x10
DB MILITARY PRESS
3x12 at 7RPE
LAT PULLDOWN
4x10-12
DB LATERAL RAISES
2x12-15
DB SKULLCRUSHERS
2x12-15
DB HAMMER CURLS
2x12-15

## WEDNESDAY

DEADLIFT
77.5%x8, 70%x3x8
BOX DEADLIFT
3x12 at 7RPE
BELT SQUAT
2x15
BACK RAISES
3x10

## THURSDAY

OFF

## FRIDAY

SQUAT
70-75%x5x8
LEG PRESS
3x10-12 at 7RPE
BOX DEADLIFT
3x12 at 6RPE
GHR
3x10

## SATURDAY

INCLINE BENCH
70-75%x5x10
CHEST PRESS
3x12 at 7RPE
CABLE ROWS
4x10-12
TRICEP PUSHDOWNS
2x12-15
DB FRONT RAISES
2x12-15
EZ BAR CURLS
2x12-15

# HYPERTROPHY BLOCK
# WEEK 2

## MONDAY

HIGH BAR SQUAT
67-72%x5x8
FRONT SQUAT
72-77%x4x8
SPLIT SQUAT
3x10 each leg
HAMSTRING CURLS
3x12

## TUESDAY

BENCH
80%x10, 70-72.5%x4x10
DB MILITARY PRESS
4x12 at 7-8RPE
LAT PULLDOWN
5x10-12
DB LATERAL RAISES
2-3x12-15
DB SKULLCRUSHERS
2-3x12-15
DB HAMMER CURLS
2-3x12-15

## WEDNESDAY

3" BLOCK PULL
70-75%x5x8
BOX DEADLIFT
4x12 at 7-8RPE
BELT SQUAT
2x15
BACK RAISES
4x10

## THURSDAY

OFF

## FRIDAY

SQUAT
90%x1, 80%x8, 67.5-72.5%x2x8
LEG PRESS
4x10-12 at 8RPE
BOX DEADLIFT
3x12 at 7RPE
GHR
3x12

## SATURDAY

INCLINE BENCH
72-77%x6x10
CHEST PRESS
4x12 at 7RPE
CABLE ROWS
5x10-12
TRICEP PUSHDOWNS
2-3x12-15
DB FRONT RAISES
2-3x12-15
EZ BAR CURLS
2-3x12-15

# HYPERTROPHY BLOCK
# WEEK 3

## MONDAY

HIGH BAR SQUAT
68-73%x5x6
FRONT SQUAT
73-78%x4x6
SPLIT SQUAT
3x8 each leg
HAMSTRING CURLS
3x15

## TUESDAY

WIDEGRIP BENCH
73-78%x7x8
DB MILITARY PRESS
4x10 at 7RPE
LAT PULLDOWN
5x10-12
DB LATERAL RAISES
3x12-15
DB SKULLCRUSHERS
3x12-15
DB HAMMER CURLS
3x12-15

## WEDNESDAY

DEADLIFT
83%x6, 73%x4x6
BOX DEADLIFT
4x10 at 7-8RPE
BELT SQUAT
2x12
BACK RAISES
5x10

## THURSDAY

OFF

## FRIDAY

SQUAT
78-82%x6x6
LEG PRESS
4x8-10 at 7RPE
BOX DEADLIFT
3x10 at 6-7RPE
GHR
3x15

## SATURDAY

INCLINE BENCH
73-78%x6x8
CHEST PRESS
4x10 at 7RPE
CABLE ROWS
5x10-12
TRICEP PUSHDOWNS
3x12-15
DB FRONT RAISES
3x12-15
EZ BAR CURLS
3x12-15

# HYPERTROPHY BLOCK
# WEEK 4

## MONDAY

HIGH BAR SQUAT
70-75%x6x6
FRONT SQUAT
75-80%x5x6
SPLIT SQUAT
4x8 each leg
HAMSTRING CURLS
3x18

## TUESDAY

BENCH
85%x8, 73-76%x4x8
DB MILITARY PRESS
5x10 at 7-8RPE
LAT PULLDOWN
6x10-12
DB LATERAL RAISES
3-4x12-15
DB SKULLCRUSHERS
3-4x12-15
DB HAMMER CURLS
3-4x12-15

## WEDNESDAY

3" BLOCK PULL
73-78%x6x6
BOX DEADLIFT
5x10 at 8RPE
BELT SQUAT
2x12
BACK RAISES
6x10

## THURSDAY

OFF

## FRIDAY

SQUAT
92%x1, 86%x6, 70-75%x3x6
LEG PRESS
5x8-10 at 8RPE
BOX DEADLIFT
3x10 at 7RPE
GHR
3x18

## SATURDAY

INCLINE BENCH
75-80%x7x8
CHEST PRESS
5x10 at 8RPE
CABLE ROWS
6x10-12
TRICEP PUSHDOWNS
3-4x12-15
DB FRONT RAISES
3-4x12-15
EZ BAR CURLS
3-4x12-15

# HYPERTROPHY BLOCK
# DELOAD

## MONDAY

HIGH BAR SQUAT
60-65%x4x6
FRONT SQUAT
65-70%x2x6
SPLIT SQUAT
2x8 each leg
HAMSTRING CURLS
2x15

## TUESDAY

BENCH
65-70%x3x8
DB MILITARY PRESS
3x10 at 7RPE
LAT PULLDOWN
4x10-12
DB LATERAL RAISES
2x12-15
DB SKULLCRUSHERS
2x12-15
DB HAMMER CURLS
2x12-15

## WEDNESDAY

DEADLIFT
65%x4x6
BOX DEADLIFT
3x10 at 6-7RPE
BELT SQUAT
2x12
BACK RAISES
4x10

## THURSDAY

OFF

## FRIDAY

SQUAT
65-70%x4x6
LEG PRESS
3x8-10 at 7RPE
BOX DEADLIFT
3x10 at 6-7RPE
GHR
2x15

## SATURDAY

INCLINE BENCH
70%x4x8
CHEST PRESS
3x10 at 7RPE
CABLE ROWS
4x10-12
TRICEP PUSHDOWNS
2x12-15
DB FRONT RAISES
2x12-15
EZ BAR CURLS
2x12-15

# STRENGTH BLOCK
# WEEK 6

## MONDAY

HIGH BAR SQUAT
72-77%x5x5
FRONT SQUAT
77-82%x3x5
SPLIT SQUAT
3x8 each leg
HAMSTRING CURLS
3x12

## TUESDAY

WIDEGRIP BENCH
75-80%x5x6
SPOTO PRESS
73-78%x3x6
LAT PULLDOWNS
5x8-10
DB LATERAL RAISES
3x10-12
DB SKULLCRUSHERS
3x10-12
DB HAMMER CURLS
3x10-12

## WEDNESDAY

DEADLIFT
88%x5, 76%x3x5
BOX DEADLIFT
4x8 at 7RPE
BACK RAISES
4x12

## THURSDAY

OFF

## FRIDAY

SQUAT
81-84%x5x5
LEG PRESS
4x8 at 7RPE
DEADLIFT
65-70%x3x5
GHR
3x10

## SATURDAY

INCLINE BENCH
77-82%x5x6
DB MILITARY PRESS
3x8 at 7RPE
CABLE ROWS
5x8-10
TRICEP PUSHDOWNS
3x10-12
DB FRONT RAISES
3x10-12
EZ BAR CURLS
3x10-12

# STRENGTH BLOCK
# WEEK 7

## MONDAY

HIGH BAR SQUAT
75-80%x4x5
FRONT SQUAT
80-85%x2x5
SPLIT SQUAT
3x8 each leg
HAMSTRING CURLS
3x10

## TUESDAY

BENCH
88%x6, 76-80%x4x6
LAT PULLDOWNS
5x8-10
DB LATERAL RAISES
3x10-12
DB SKULLCRUSHERS
3x10-12
DB HAMMER CURLS
3x10-12

## WEDNESDAY

3" BLOCK PULL
76-80%x5x5
BOX DEADLIFT
4x8 at 8RPE
BACK RAISES
4x10

## THURSDAY

OFF

## FRIDAY

SQUAT
94%x1, 89%x5, 73-78%x2x5
LEG PRESS
4x8 at 8RPE
DEADLIFT
67-72%x3x4
GHR
3x10

## SATURDAY

INCLINE BENCH
80-85%x4x6
DB MILITARY PRESS
3x8 at 7RPE
CABLE ROWS
5x8-10
TRICEP PUSHDOWNS
3x10-12
DB FRONT RAISES
3x10-12
EZ BAR CURLS
3x10-12

# STRENGTH BLOCK
# WEEK 8

## MONDAY

HIGH BAR SQUAT
78-83%x5x4
FRONT SQUAT
83-88%x3x4
SPLIT SQUAT
3x6 each leg
HAMSTRING CURLS
3x10

## TUESDAY

WIDEGRIP BENCH
78-83%x5x5
SPOTO PRESS
75-80%x3x5
LAT PULLDOWNS
5x8-10
DB LATERAL RAISES
3x10-12
DB SKULLCRUSHERS
3x10-12
DB HAMMER CURLS
3x10-12

## WEDNESDAY

DEADLIFT
90%x3, 82%x3x3
BOX DEADLIFT
4x6 at 7-8RPE
BACK RAISES
4x8

## THURSDAY

OFF

## FRIDAY

SQUAT
83-87%x5x4
LEG PRESS
4x6 at 7RPE
DEADLIFT
70-75%x3x3
GHR
3x10

## SATURDAY

INCLINE BENCH
82-87%x5x5
DB MILITARY PRESS
3x6 at 7RPE
CABLE ROWS
5x8-10
TRICEP PUSHDOWNS
3x10-12
DB FRONT RAISES
3x10-12
EZ BAR CURLS
3x10-12

# STRENGTH BLOCK
# WEEK 9

## MONDAY

HIGH BAR SQUAT
80-85%x4x4
FRONT SQUAT
85-90%x2x4
SPLIT SQUAT
3x6 each leg
HAMSTRING CURLS
3x10

## TUESDAY

BENCH
91%x5, 79-83%x4x5
LAT PULLDOWNS
5x8-10
DB LATERAL RAISES
3x10-12
DB SKULLCRUSHERS
3x10-12
DB HAMMER CURLS
3x10-12

## WEDNESDAY

3" BLOCK PULL
79-83%x5x3
BOX DEADLIFT
4x6 at 8RPE
BACK RAISES
4x6

## THURSDAY

OFF

## FRIDAY

SQUAT
97%x1, 92%x4, 76-81%x2x4
LEG PRESS
4x6 at 8RPE
DEADLIFT
72-77%x3x3
GHR
3x10

## SATURDAY

INCLINE BENCH
84-89%x4x5
DB MILITARY PRESS
3x6 at 8RPE
CABLE ROWS
5x8-10
TRICEP PUSHDOWNS
3x10-12
DB FRONT RAISES
3x10-12
EZ BAR CURLS
3x10-12

# STRENGTH BLOCK
# DELOAD

## MONDAY

HIGH BAR SQUAT
65-70%x3x4
FRONT SQUAT
70-75%x2x4
SPLIT SQUAT
3x6 each leg
HAMSTRING CURLS
3x10

## TUESDAY

BENCH
65-70%x4x5
LAT PULLDOWNS
4x8-10
DB LATERAL RAISES
2x10-12
DB SKULLCRUSHERS
2x10-12
DB HAMMER CURLS
2x10-12

## WEDNESDAY

DEADLIFT
70%x3x5
BOX DEADLIFT
3x6 at 6RPE
BACK RAISES
3x8

## THURSDAY

OFF

## FRIDAY

SQUAT
70-75%x3x4
LEG PRESS
2x6 at 7RPE
DEADLIFT
60%x2x3
GHR
3x10

## SATURDAY

INCLINE BENCH
75%x3x5
DB MILITARY PRESS
2x6 at 7RPE
CABLE ROWS
4x8-10
TRICEP PUSHDOWNS
2x10-12
DB FRONT RAISES
2x10-12
EZ BAR CURLS
2x10-12

# PEAKING BLOCK
# WEEK 11

| MONDAY | TUESDAY | WEDNESDAY |
|---|---|---|
| DEADLIFT | OFF | BENCH |
| 85/91/97%x1 | | 101%x1, 87%x5x3 |
| SQUAT | | SQUAT |
| 93%x1, 88%x3x2 | | 87%x1, 80%x3x3 |
| BENCH | | LAT PULLDOWNS |
| 94%x1, 86%x3x2 | | 4x6-8 |
| | | DB LATERAL RAISES |
| | | 2-3x8-10 |
| | | DB SKULLCRUSHERS |
| | | 2-3x8-10 |
| | | DB HAMMER CURLS |
| | | 2-3x8-10 |

| THURSDAY | FRIDAY | SATURDAY |
|---|---|---|
| OFF | SQUAT | WIDEGRIP BENCH |
| | 87/94/101%x1, 90%x3x2 | 80%x3x5 |
| | DEADLIFT | INCLINE BENCH |
| | 70%x3-5x1 | 80%x3x5 |
| | GHR | CABLE ROWS |
| | 3x8-10 | 3x8-10 |
| | | TRICEP PUSHDOWNS |
| | | 2x10-12 |
| | | DB FRONT RAISES |
| | | 2x10-12 |
| | | EZ BAR CURLS |
| | | 2x10-12 |

# PEAKING BLOCK
# WEEK 12

## MONDAY

DEADLIFT
80%x5x1
SQUAT
95%x1, 90%x2x2
BENCH
97%x1, 88%x2x2

## TUESDAY

OFF

## WEDNESDAY

BENCH
102%x1, 91%x4x2
SQUAT
89%x1, 82%x2x3
LAT PULLDOWNS
4x6-8
DB LATERAL RAISES
2-3x8-10
DB SKULLCRUSHERS
2-3x8-10
DB HAMMER CURLS
2-3x8-10

## THURSDAY

OFF

## FRIDAY

SQUAT
89/96/102%x1, 92%x2x2
DEADLIFT
70%x3-5x1
GHR
3x8-10

## SATURDAY

WIDEGRIP BENCH
83%x3x4
INCLINE BENCH
83%x3x4
CABLE ROWS
3x8-10
TRICEP PUSHDOWNS
2x10-12
DB FRONT RAISES
2x10-12
EZ BAR CURLS
2x10-12

# PEAKING BLOCK
# WEEK 13

## MONDAY

DEADLIFT
80/85/90%x1
SQUAT
90%x1, 85%x3
BENCH
101%x1, 85%x2

## TUESDAY

OFF

## WEDNESDAY

BENCH
92/97/103%x1, 95%x2
SQUAT
102%x1, 95%x3x1
LAT PULLDOWNS
4x6-8
DB LATERAL RAISES
2-3x8-10
DB SKULLCRUSHERS
2-3x8-10
DB HAMMER CURLS
2-3x8-10

## THURSDAY

OFF

## FRIDAY

SQUAT
88%x1, 80%x2x2
DEADLIFT
70%x3-5x1
GHR
3x8-10

## SATURDAY

WIDEGRIP BENCH
86%x3x3
INCLINE BENCH
86%x3x3
CABLE ROWS
3x8-10
TRICEP PUSHDOWNS
2x10-12
DB FRONT RAISES
2x10-12
EZ BAR CURLS
2x10-12

# PEAKING BLOCK
# MEET WEEK

## MONDAY

DEADLIFT
83%x1, 75%x2x3
SQUAT
92%x1, 80%x3x3
BENCH
67%x3x1

## TUESDAY

OFF

## WEDNESDAY

SQUAT
72-78%x3x1
BENCH
85%x1, 72%x2x3
DEADLIFT
60%x3x1

## THURSDAY

OFF

## FRIDAY

LIGHT WARMUP

## SATURDAY

COMPETE

# PHYSIQUE PROGRAM

In this program, we aim to attack bodypart by bodypart with high volume, submaximal intensity training to build muscle in a balanced physique. This program will challenge your work capacity and create new hypertrophy throughout your body. If you'd like to, you can add in Cardio 2-3x/week following the different guidelines laid out in the Cardio section of the book. When exercises are listed as 2A, 2B, those exercises are to be performed as a SuperSet or Circuit.

## HOW TO PERFORM DROP SETS:

Start with the heaviest weight for the lowest listed reps, perform reps, immediately upon completion, drop weight and begin next rep range, drop weight again and complete final rep range. For example:

### SET 1:

100# x8-No Rest
80# x10-No Rest
60# x12-Rest 1 to 3 Minutes

### SET 2:

100# x8-No Rest
80# x10-No Rest
60# x12-Rest 1 to 3 Minutes

### SET 3:

100# x8-No Rest
80# x10-No Rest
60# x12-Rest 1 to 3 Minutes

# PHASE 1 / WEEK 1

### DAY 1:
LEGS

1) HIGH BAR SQUAT
60%x3x12
2a) LEG PRESS
3x10 at 7RPE
2b) LUNGES
3x10 each leg
3) LEG EXTENSIONS
Drop Set: 3(8+10+12)
4) RDL
3x10 at 7RPE
5) CALF RAISES
4x15

### DAY 2: CHEST / TRICEPS / SHOULDERS

1) BENCH PRESS-FEET UP
60%x3x12
2) CHEST PRESS (Machine)
3x10 at 7RPE
3a) DB LATERAL RAISES
3x10 at 7RPE
3b) DB FRONT RAISES
3x10 at 7RPE
4a) MILITARY PUSHUPS
3x10 at 7RPE
4b) TRICEP PUSHDOWNS
3x10 at 7RPE
4c) FACE PULLS
3x10 at 7RPE

### DAY 3:
BACK / BICEPS

1) RACK / BLOCK PULLS FROM BELOW KNEE
60%x3x12
2) LAT PULLDOWNS
3x10 at 7RPE
3) BENTOVER ROWS
4x10 at 7RPE
2 Sets Overhand, 2 Sets Underhand
4) CHIN-UPS
(Assisted / Weighted if Possible)
10, 10, 8
5) BACK RAISES
3x10 at 7RPE
6) DB CURLS
Drop Set: 3(8+10+12)
7) HANGING LEG RAISES
4x15

### DAY 4:
OFF

### DAY 5:
LEGS / BACK

1) FRONT SQUAT
60%x3x12
2) 1-1/2 REP LEG PRESS (All the way down, halfway up, back down, all the way up)
3x10 at 7RPE
3) REAR FOOT ELEVATED SPLIT SQUAT
3x10 at 7RPE
4) HAMSTRING CURLS OR GHRS
3x10 at 7RPE
5) PENDLAY ROWS
3x10 at 7RPE
6) CALF RAISES
4x15

### DAY 6: CHEST / TRICEPS / SHOULDERS

1) INCLINE BENCH
60%x3x12
2) CABLE CROSSOVERS
3x10 at 7RPE
3) PALMS IN DB BENCH
3x10 at 7RPE
4) DB MILITARY PRESS
3x10 at 7RPE
5) FRONT PLATE RAISES
3x10 at 7RPE
6) SEATED BENTOVER DB LATERAL RAISES
3x10 at 7RPE

### DAY 7:
OFF

# PHASE 1 / WEEK 2

## DAY 1:
### LEGS

1) HIGH BAR SQUAT
63%x3x12
2a) LEG PRESS
3x10 at 7RPE
2b) LUNGES
3x10 each leg
3) LEG EXTENSIONS
Drop Set: 3(8+10+12)
4) RDL
3x10 at 7RPE
5) CALF RAISES
4x15

## DAY 2: CHEST / TRICEPS / SHOULDERS

1) BENCH PRESS-FEET UP
63%x3x12
2) CHEST PRESS (Machine)
3x10 at 7RPE
3a) DB LATERAL RAISES
3x10 at 7RPE
3b) DB FRONT RAISES
3x10 at 7RPE
4a) MILITARY PUSHUPS
3x10 at 7RPE
4b) TRICEP PUSHDOWNS
3x10 at 7RPE
4c) FACE PULLS
3x10 at 7RPE

## DAY 3:
### BACK / BICEPS

1) RACK / BLOCK PULLS FROM BELOW KNEE
63%x3x12
2) LAT PULLDOWNS
3x10 at 7RPE
3) BENTOVER ROWS
4x10 at 7RPE
2 Sets Overhand, 2 Sets Underhand
4) CHIN-UPS
(Assisted / Weighted if Possible)
10, 10, 8
5) BACK RAISES
3x10 at 7RPE
6) DB CURLS
Drop Set: 3(8+10+12)
7) HANGING LEG RAISES
4x15

## DAY 4:
### OFF

## DAY 5:
### LEGS / BACK

1) FRONT SQUAT
63%x3x12
2) 1-1/2 REP LEG PRESS (All the way down, halfway up, back down, all the way up)
3x10 at 7RPE
3) REAR FOOT ELEVATED SPLIT SQUAT
3x10 at 7RPE
4) HAMSTRING CURLS OR GHRS
3x10 at 7RPE
5) PENDLAY ROWS
3x10 at 7RPE
6) CALF RAISES
4x15

## DAY 6: CHEST / TRICEPS / SHOULDERS

1) INCLINE BENCH
63%x3x12
2) CABLE CROSSOVERS
3x10 at 7RPE
3) PALMS IN DB BENCH
3x10 at 7RPE
4) DB MILITARY PRESS
3x10 at 7RPE
5) FRONT PLATE RAISES
3x10 at 7RPE
6) SEATED BENTOVER DB LATERAL RAISES
3x10 at 7RPE

## DAY 7:
### OFF

# PHASE 1 / WEEK 3

## DAY 1:
LEGS

1) HIGH BAR SQUAT
65%x3x10
2a) LEG PRESS
3x10 at 7.5RPE
2b) LUNGES
3x10 each leg
3) LEG EXTENSIONS
Drop Set: 3(10+10+12)
4) RDL
3x10 at 7.5RPE
5) CALF RAISES
4x15

## DAY 2: CHEST / TRICEPS / SHOULDERS

1) BENCH PRESS-FEET UP
65%x3x10
2) CHEST PRESS (Machine)
4x10 at 7.5RPE
3a) DB LATERAL RAISES
4x10 at 7.5RPE
3b) DB FRONT RAISES
3x10 at 7.5RPE
4a) MILITARY PUSHUPS
3x10 at 7.5RPE
4b) TRICEP PUSHDOWNS
3x10 at 7.5RPE
4c) FACE PULLS
3x10 at 7.5RPE

## DAY 3: BACK / BICEPS

1) RACK / BLOCK PULLS FROM BELOW KNEE
65%x3x10
2) LAT PULLDOWNS
4x10 at 7.5RPE
3) BENTOVER ROWS
4x10 at 7RPE
2 Sets Overhand, 2 Sets Underhand
4) CHIN-UPS
(Assisted / Weighted if Possible)
12, 10, 8
5) BACK RAISES
4x10 at 8RPE
6) DB CURLS
Drop Set: 3(10+10+12)
7) HANGING LEG RAISES
4x15

## DAY 4:
OFF

## DAY 5:
LEGS / BACK

1) FRONT SQUAT
65%x3x10
2) 1-1/2 REP LEG PRESS (All the way down, halfway up, back down, all the way up)
4x10 at 7.5RPE
3) REAR FOOT ELEVATED SPLIT SQUAT
4x10 at 7.5RPE
4) HAMSTRING CURLS OR GHRS
4x10 at 7.5RPE
5) PENDLAY ROWS
4x10 at 7.5RPE
6) CALF RAISES
4x15

## DAY 6: CHEST / TRICEPS / SHOULDERS

1) INCLINE BENCH
65%x3x10
2) CABLE CROSSOVERS
4x10 at 7.5RPE
3) PALMS IN DB BENCH
4x10 at 7.5RPE
4) DB MILITARY PRESS
4x10 at 7.5RPE
5) FRONT PLATE RAISES
4x10 at 7.5RPE
6) SEATED BENTOVER DB LATERAL RAISES
4x10 at 7.5RPE

## DAY 7:
OFF

# PHASE 1 / WEEK 4

## DAY 1:
### LEGS

1) HIGH BAR SQUAT
68%x3x10
2a) LEG PRESS
3x10 at 8RPE
2b) LUNGES
3x10 each leg
3) LEG EXTENSIONS
Drop Set: 3(10+10+12)
4) RDL
3x10 at 8RPE
5) CALF RAISES
4x15

## DAY 2: CHEST /
### TRICEPS / SHOULDERS

1) BENCH PRESS-FEET UP
68%x3x10
2) CHEST PRESS (Machine)
4x10 at 8RPE
3a) DB LATERAL RAISES
4x10 at 8RPE
3b) DB FRONT RAISES
3x10 at 8RPE
4a) MILITARY PUSHUPS
3x10 at 8RPE
4b) TRICEP PUSHDOWNS
3x10 at 8RPE
4c) FACE PULLS
3x10 at 8RPE

## DAY 3:
### BACK / BICEPS

1) RACK / BLOCK PULLS
FROM BELOW KNEE
68%x3x10
2) LAT PULLDOWNS
4x10 at 8RPE
3) BENTOVER ROWS
4x10 at 8RPE
2 Sets Overhand, 2 Sets Underhand
4) CHIN-UPS
(Assisted / Weighted if Possible)
12, 10, 8
5) BACK RAISES
4x10 at 8RPE
6) DB CURLS
Drop Set: 3(10+10+12)
7) HANGING LEG RAISES
4x15

## DAY 4:
### OFF

## DAY 5:
### LEGS / BACK

1) FRONT SQUAT
68%x3x10
2) 1-1/2 REP LEG PRESS (All the way down,
halfway up, back down, all the way up)
4x10 at 8RPE
3) REAR FOOT ELEVATED SPLIT SQUAT
4x10 at 8RPE
4) HAMSTRING CURLS OR GHRS
4x10 at 8RPE
5) PENDLAY ROWS
4x10 at 8RPE
6) CALF RAISES
4x15

## DAY 6: CHEST /
### TRICEPS / SHOULDERS

1) INCLINE BENCH
68%x3x10
2) CABLE CROSSOVERS
4x10 at 8RPE
3) PALMS IN DB BENCH
4x10 at 8RPE
4) DB MILITARY PRESS
4x10 at 8RPE
5) FRONT PLATE RAISES
4x10 at 8RPE
6) SEATED BENTOVER DB
LATERAL RAISES
4x10 at 8RPE

## DAY 7:
### OFF

# PHASE 1 / WEEK 5

**DAY 1:**
LEGS

1) HIGH BAR SQUAT
70%x3x8
2a) LEG PRESS
3x10 at 8RPE
2b) LUNGES
3x10 each leg
3) LEG EXTENSIONS
Drop Set: 3(10+10+12)
4) RDL
3x10 at 8RPE
5) CALF RAISES
4x15

**DAY 2:** CHEST /
TRICEPS / SHOULDERS

1) BENCH PRESS-FEET UP
70%x3x8
2) CHEST PRESS (Machine)
4x10 at 8RPE
3a) DB LATERAL RAISES
4x10 at 8RPE
3b) DB FRONT RAISES
3x10 at 8RPE
4a) MILITARY PUSHUPS
3x10 at 8RPE
4b) TRICEP PUSHDOWNS
3x10 at 8RPE
4c) FACE PULLS
3x10 at 8RPE

**DAY 3:**
BACK / BICEPS

1) RACK / BLOCK PULLS
FROM BELOW KNEE
70%x3x8
2) LAT PULLDOWNS
4x10 at 8RPE
3) BENTOVER ROWS
4x10 at 8RPE
2 Sets Overhand, 2 Sets Underhand
4) CHIN-UPS
(Assisted / Weighted if Possible)
12, 10, 10
5) BACK RAISES
4x10 at 8RPE
6) DB CURLS
Drop Set: 3(10+10+12)
7) HANGING LEG RAISES
4x15

**DAY 4:**
OFF

**DAY 5:**
LEGS / BACK

1) FRONT SQUAT
70%x3x8
2) 1-1/2 REP LEG PRESS (All the way down,
halfway up, back down, all the way up)
4x10 at 8RPE
3) REAR FOOT ELEVATED SPLIT SQUAT
4x10 at 8RPE
4) HAMSTRING CURLS OR GHRS
4x10 at 8RPE
5) PENDLAY ROWS
4x10 at 8RPE
6) CALF RAISES
4x15

**DAY 6:** CHEST /
TRICEPS / SHOULDERS

1) INCLINE BENCH
70%x3x8
2) CABLE CROSSOVERS
4x10 at 8RPE
3) PALMS IN DB BENCH
4x10 at 8RPE
4) DB MILITARY PRESS
4x10 at 8RPE
5) FRONT PLATE RAISES
4x10 at 8RPE
6) SEATED BENTOVER DB
LATERAL RAISES
4x10 at 8RPE

**DAY 7:**
OFF

# PHASE 1 / DELOAD

## DAY 1:
### LEGS

1) HIGH BAR SQUAT
65%x2x6

2a) LEG PRESS
2x8 at 7RPE

2b) LUNGES
2x8 each leg

3) LEG EXTENSIONS
2x8

4) RDL
2x8 at 7RPE

5) CALF RAISES
3x12

## DAY 2: CHEST / TRICEPS / SHOULDERS

1) BENCH PRESS-FEET UP
65%x2x6

2) CHEST PRESS (Machine)
3x8 at 7RPE

3a) DB LATERAL RAISES
3x8 at 7RPE

3b) DB FRONT RAISES
2x8 at 7RPE

4a) MILITARY PUSHUPS
2x8 at 7RPE

4b) TRICEP PUSHDOWNS
2x8 at 7RPE

4c) FACE PULLS
2x8 at 7RPE

## DAY 3:
### BACK / BICEPS

1) RACK / BLOCK PULLS FROM BELOW KNEE
65%x2x6

2) LAT PULLDOWNS
2x8 at 7RPE

3) BENTOVER ROWS
2x8 at 7RPE
2 Sets Overhand, 2 Sets Underhand

4) CHIN-UPS
(Assisted / Weighted if Possible)
8, 6, 6

5) BACK RAISES
2x8 at 7RPE

6) DB CURLS
2x8

7) HANGING LEG RAISES
3x12

## DAY 4:
### OFF

## DAY 5:
### LEGS / BACK

1) FRONT SQUAT
65%x2x6

2) 1-1/2 REP LEG PRESS (All the way down, halfway up, back down, all the way up)
2x8 at 7RPE

3) REAR FOOT ELEVATED SPLIT SQUAT
2x8 at 7RPE

4) HAMSTRING CURLS OR GHRS
2x8 at 7RPE

5) PENDLAY ROWS
2x8 at 7RPE

6) CALF RAISES
3x12

## DAY 6: CHEST / TRICEPS / SHOULDERS

1) INCLINE BENCH
65%x2x6

2) CABLE CROSSOVERS
2x8 at 7RPE

3) PALMS IN DB BENCH
2x8 at 7RPE

4) DB MILITARY PRESS
2x8 at 7RPE

5) FRONT PLATE RAISES
2x8 at 7RPE

6) SEATED BENTOVER DB LATERAL RAISES
2x8 at 7RPE

## DAY 7:
### OFF

# PHASE 2 / WEEK 1

## DAY 1:
LEGS

1) HIGH BAR SQUAT
73%x3x10
2a) GOBLET SQUAT
3x10 at 7RPE
2b) STEP UPS
3x10 each leg
3) REVERSE LUNGES
3x10 at 7RPE
4) SUMO RDL
3x10 at 7RPE
5) CALF RAISES
4x15

## DAY 2: CHEST / TRICEPS / SHOULDERS

1) BENCH PRESS-FEET UP
73%x3x10
2a) DB INCLINE BENCH
3x10 at 7RPE
2b) DB INCLINE FLIES
3x10 at 7RPE
3) UPRIGHT ROWS
3x10 at 7RPE
4a) DECLINE PUSHUPS
3x10 at 7RPE
4b) DB SKULLCRUSHERS
3x10 at 7RPE
4c) BENTOVER DB LATERAL RAISES
3x10 at 7RPE

## DAY 3: BACK / BICEPS

1) RACK / BLOCK PULLS FROM BELOW KNEE
73%x3x10
2) CLOSEGRIP PULLDOWNS
3x10 at 7RPE
3) DB ROWS
3x10 at 7RPE
4) PULLUPS OR INVERTED ROWS
10, 10, 8
5) BACK RAISES
3x10 at 7RPE
6) DB 21S (7 Top Half ROM, 7 Bottom Half ROM, 7 Full ROM Curls)
3 Sets at 7RPE
7) DECLINE SITUPS
4x15

## DAY 4:
OFF

## DAY 5:
LEGS / BACK

1) FRONT SQUAT
73%x3x10
2) HACK SQUAT
3x10 at 7RPE
3) WALKING LUNGES
3x20 Steps
4) SINGLE LEG GLUTE BRIDGES
3x10 at 7RPE
5) LANDMINE ROWS
3x10 at 7RPE
6) CALF RAISES
4x15

## DAY 6: CHEST / TRICEPS / SHOULDERS

1) INCLINE BENCH
73%x3x10
2a) DB BENCH
3x10 at 7RPE
2b) DB FLIES
3x10 at 7RPE
3) TRICEP KICKBACKS
3x10 at 7RPE
4) SINGLE ARM DB OVERHEAD PRESS
3x10 at 7RPE
5a) DB FRONT RAISES
3x10 at 7RPE
5b) DB REVERSE FLIES
3x10 at 7RPE

## DAY 7:
OFF

# PHASE 2 / WEEK 2

## DAY 1:
LEGS

1) HIGH BAR SQUAT
75%x3x8
2a) GOBLET SQUAT
3x10 at 7RPE
2b) STEP UPS
3x10 each leg
3) REVERSE LUNGES
3x10 at 7RPE
4) SUMO RDL
3x10 at 7RPE
5) CALF RAISES
4x15

## DAY 2: CHEST / TRICEPS / SHOULDERS

1) BENCH PRESS-FEET UP
75%x3x8
2a) DB INCLINE BENCH
3x10 at 7RPE
2b) DB INCLINE FLIES
3x10 at 7RPE
3) UPRIGHT ROWS
3x10 at 7RPE
4a) DECLINE PUSHUPS
3x10 at 7RPE
4b) DB SKULLCRUSHERS
3x10 at 7RPE
4c) BENTOVER DB LATERAL RAISES
3x10 at 7RPE

## DAY 3:
BACK / BICEPS

1) RACK / BLOCK PULLS FROM BELOW KNEE
75%x3x8
2) CLOSEGRIP PULLDOWNS
3x10 at 7RPE
3) DB ROWS
3x10 at 7RPE
4) PULLUPS OR INVERTED ROWS
10, 10, 8
5) BACK RAISES
3x10 at 7RPE
6) DB 21S (7 Top Half ROM, 7 Bottom Half ROM, 7 Full ROM Curls)
3 Sets at 7RPE
7) DECLINE SITUPS
4x15

## DAY 4:
OFF

## DAY 5:
LEGS / BACK

1) FRONT SQUAT
75%x3x8
2) HACK SQUAT
3x10 at 7RPE
3) WALKING LUNGES
3x20 Steps
4) SINGLE LEG GLUTE BRIDGES
3x10 at 7RPE
5) LANDMINE ROWS
3x10 at 7RPE
6) CALF RAISES
4x15

## DAY 6: CHEST / TRICEPS / SHOULDERS

1) INCLINE BENCH
75%x3x8
2a) DB BENCH
3x10 at 7RPE
2b) DB FLIES
3x10 at 7RPE
3) TRICEP KICKBACKS
3x10 at 7RPE
4) SINGLE ARM DB OVERHEAD PRESS
3x10 at 7RPE
5a) DB FRONT RAISES
3x10 at 7RPE
5b) DB REVERSE FLIES
3x10 at 7RPE

## DAY 7:
OFF

# PHASE 2 / WEEK 3

## DAY 1:
### LEGS

1) HIGH BAR SQUAT
78%x3x8

2a) GOBLET SQUAT
3x10 at 7.5RPE

2b) STEP UPS
3x10 each leg

3) REVERSE LUNGES
3x10 at 7.5RPE

4) SUMO RDL
3x10 at 7.5RPE

5) CALF RAISES
4x15

## DAY 2: CHEST / TRICEPS / SHOULDERS

1) BENCH PRESS-FEET UP
78%x3x8

2a) DB INCLINE BENCH
4x10 at 7.5RPE

2b) DB INCLINE FLIES
4x10 at 7.5RPE

3) UPRIGHT ROWS
4x10 at 7.5RPE

4a) DECLINE PUSHUPS
4x10 at 7.5RPE

4b) DB SKULLCRUSHERS
4x10 at 7.5RPE

4c) BENTOVER DB
LATERAL RAISES
4x10 at 7.5RPE

## DAY 3:
### BACK / BICEPS

1) RACK / BLOCK PULLS
FROM BELOW KNEE
78%x3x8

2) CLOSEGRIP PULLDOWNS
4x10 at 7.5RPE

3) DB ROWS
4x10 at 7.5RPE

4) PULLUPS OR INVERTED ROWS
12, 10, 8

5) BACK RAISES
4x10 at 8RPE

6) DB 21S [7 Top Half ROM, 7 Bottom Half ROM, 7 Full ROM Curls]
4 Sets at 7.5RPE

7) DECLINE SITUPS
4x15

## DAY 4:
### OFF

## DAY 5:
### LEGS / BACK

1) FRONT SQUAT
78%x3x8

2) HACK SQUAT
4x10 at 7.5RPE

3) WALKING LUNGES
4x20 Steps

4) SINGLE LEG GLUTE BRIDGES
4x10 at 7.5RPE

5) LANDMINE ROWS
4x10 at 7.5RPE

6) CALF RAISES
4x15

## DAY 6: CHEST / TRICEPS / SHOULDERS

1) INCLINE BENCH
78%x3x8

2a) DB BENCH
4x10 at 7.5RPE

2b) DB FLIES
4x10 at 7.5RPE

3) TRICEP KICKBACKS
4x10 at 7.5RPE

4) SINGLE ARM DB
OVERHEAD PRESS
4x10 at 7.5RPE

5a) DB FRONT RAISES
4x10 at 7.5RPE

5b) DB REVERSE FLIES
4x10 at 7.5RPE

## DAY 7:
### OFF

# PHASE 2 / WEEK 4

## DAY 1:
LEGS

1) HIGH BAR SQUAT
80%x3x6
2a) GOBLET SQUAT
3x10 at 8RPE
2b) STEP UPS
3x10 each leg
3) REVERSE LUNGES
3x10 at 8RPE
4) SUMO RDL
3x10 at 8RPE
5) CALF RAISES
4x15

## DAY 2: CHEST /
TRICEPS / SHOULDERS

1) BENCH PRESS-FEET UP
80%x3x6
2a) DB INCLINE BENCH
4x10 at 8RPE
2b) DB INCLINE FLIES
4x10 at 8RPE
3) UPRIGHT ROWS
3x10 at 8RPE
4a) DECLINE PUSHUPS
3x10 at 8RPE
4b) DB SKULLCRUSHERS
3x10 at 8RPE
4c) BENTOVER DB
LATERAL RAISES
3x10 at 8RPE

## DAY 3:
BACK / BICEPS

1) RACK / BLOCK PULLS
FROM BELOW KNEE
80%x3x6
2) CLOSEGRIP PULLDOWNS
4x10 at 8RPE
3) DB ROWS
4x10 at 8RPE
4) PULLUPS OR INVERTED ROWS
12, 10, 8
5) BACK RAISES
4x10 at 8RPE
6) DB 21S (7 Top Half ROM, 7 Bottom
Half ROM, 7 Full ROM Curls)
4 Sets at 8RPE
7) DECLINE SITUPS
4x15

## DAY 4:
OFF

## DAY 5:
LEGS / BACK

1) FRONT SQUAT
80%x3x6
2) HACK SQUAT
4x10 at 8RPE
3) WALKING LUNGES
4x20 Steps
4) SINGLE LEG GLUTE BRIDGES
4x10 at 8RPE
5) LANDMINE ROWS
4x10 at 8RPE
6) CALF RAISES
4x15

## DAY 6: CHEST /
TRICEPS / SHOULDERS

1) INCLINE BENCH
80%x3x6
2a) DB BENCH
4x10 at 8RPE
2b) DB FLIES
4x10 at 8RPE
3) TRICEP KICKBACKS
4x10 at 8RPE
4) SINGLE ARM DB
OVERHEAD PRESS
4x10 at 8RPE
5a) DB FRONT RAISES
4x10 at 8RPE
5b) DB REVERSE FLIES
4x10 at 8RPE

## DAY 7:
OFF

# PHASE 2 / WEEK 5

### DAY 1:
LEGS

1) HIGH BAR SQUAT
83%x3x6

2a) GOBLET SQUAT
3x10 at 8RPE

2b) STEP UPS
3x10 each leg

3) REVERSE LUNGES
3x10 at 8RPE

4) SUMO RDL
3x10 at 8RPE

5) CALF RAISES
4x15

### DAY 2: CHEST / TRICEPS / SHOULDERS

1) BENCH PRESS-FEET UP
83%x3x6

2a) DB INCLINE BENCH
4x10 at 8RPE

2b) DB INCLINE FLIES
4x10 at 8RPE

3) UPRIGHT ROWS
3x10 at 8RPE

4a) DECLINE PUSHUPS
3x10 at 8RPE

4b) DB SKULLCRUSHERS
3x10 at 8RPE

4c) BENTOVER DB LATERAL RAISES
3x10 at 8RPE

### DAY 3:
BACK / BICEPS

1) RACK / BLOCK PULLS FROM BELOW KNEE
83%x3x6

2) CLOSEGRIP PULLDOWNS
4x10 at 8RPE

3) DB ROWS
4x10 at 8RPE

4) PULLUPS OR INVERTED ROWS
12, 10, 10

5) BACK RAISES
4x10 at 8RPE

6) DB 21S (7 Top Half ROM, 7 Bottom Half ROM, 7 Full ROM Curls)
4 Sets at 8RPE

7) DECLINE SITUPS
4x15

### DAY 4:
OFF

### DAY 5:
LEGS / BACK

1) FRONT SQUAT
83%x3x6

2) HACK SQUAT
4x10 at 8RPE

3) WALKING LUNGES
4x20 Steps

4) SINGLE LEG GLUTE BRIDGES
4x10 at 8RPE

5) LANDMINE ROWS
4x10 at 8RPE

6) CALF RAISES
4x15

### DAY 6: CHEST / TRICEPS / SHOULDERS

1) INCLINE BENCH
83%x3x6

2a) DB BENCH
4x10 at 8RPE

2b) DB FLIES
4x10 at 8RPE

3) TRICEP KICKBACKS
4x10 at 8RPE

4) SINGLE ARM DB OVERHEAD PRESS
4x10 at 8RPE

5a) DB FRONT RAISES
4x10 at 8RPE

5b) DB REVERSE FLIES
4x10 at 8RPE

### DAY 7:
OFF

# PHASE 2 / DELOAD

### DAY 1:
LEGS

1) HIGH BAR SQUAT
65%x2x6

2a) GOBLET SQUAT
2x8 at 7RPE

2b) STEP UPS
2x8 each leg

3) REVERSE LUNGES
2x8 at 7RPE

4) SUMO RDL
2x8 at 7RPE

5) CALF RAISES
3x12

### DAY 2: CHEST / TRICEPS / SHOULDERS

1) BENCH PRESS-FEET UP
65%x2x6

2a) DB INCLINE BENCH
3x8 at 7RPE

2b) DB INCLINE FLIES
3x8 at 7RPE

3) UPRIGHT ROWS
2x8 at 7RPE

4a) DECLINE PUSHUPS
2x8 at 7RPE

4b) DB SKULLCRUSHERS
2x8 at 7RPE

4c) BENTOVER DB LATERAL RAISES
2x8 at 7RPE

### DAY 3:
BACK / BICEPS

1) RACK / BLOCK PULLS FROM BELOW KNEE
65%x2x6

2) CLOSEGRIP PULLDOWNS
2x8 at 7RPE

3) DB ROWS
2x8 at 7RPE

4) PULLUPS OR INVERTED ROWS
8, 6, 6

5) BACK RAISES
2x8 at 7RPE

6) DB 21S (7 Top Half ROM, 7 Bottom Half ROM, 7 Full ROM Curls)
2x8

7) DECLINE SITUPS
3x12

### DAY 4:
OFF

### DAY 5:
LEGS / BACK

1) FRONT SQUAT
65%x2x6

2) HACK SQUAT
2x8 at 7RPE

3) WALKING LUNGES
2x16 Steps

4) SINGLE LEG GLUTE BRIDGES
2x8 at 7RPE

5) LANDMINE ROWS
2x8 at 7RPE

6) CALF RAISES
3x12

### DAY 6: CHEST / TRICEPS / SHOULDERS

1) INCLINE BENCH
65%x2x6

2a) DB BENCH
2x8 at 7RPE

2b) DB FLIES
2x8 at 7RPE

3) TRICEP KICKBACKS
2x8 at 7RPE

4) SINGLE ARM DB OVERHEAD PRESS
2x8 at 7RPE

5a) DB FRONT RAISES
2x8 at 7RPE

5b) DB REVERSE FLIES
2x8 at 7RPE

### DAY 7:
OFF